I0104202

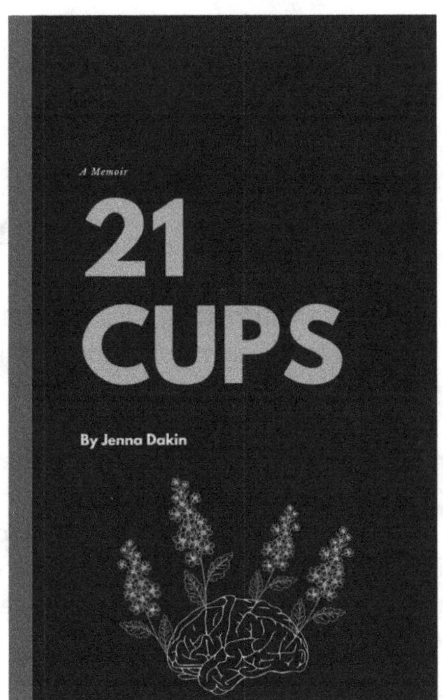
A Memoir
21 CUPS
By Jenna Dakin

21 Cups

www.21-cups.com
ISBN: 978-1-990330-34-6

Cover design: Jenna Dakin

Editing and formatting: Lisa Browning
One Thousand Trees - www.onethousandtrees.com

"Will you take me as I am? Will you?"

Joni Mitchell, *California*

Acknowledgements

Thank you to all my readers, I appreciate you. Thank you to all my supporters who have been, and continue to be there for me. I appreciate you.

Thank you to my publisher Lisa, who immediately jumped on board and made this a reality. Who consistently reassured me I can do this and that I'm actually pretty cool.

To Jordan, the one who I never forgot. Thank you for never treating me any differently, for remaining my sibling. For being there for Mom, for me, and for always being you. I'm so proud of you and honour your bravery on this new adventure of your life.

To Mom, my core support. Thank you for showing up every single day. For pushing past the limits of exhaustion, stress, and I can't even imagine what else to be there with me, thank you. You advocate your heart out, your love is unconditional, and you have helped me create myself again. I cannot wait for our future adventures together, maybe even one in a real ocean.

To Pat, I'm unsure where to begin. I don't know many other people who would have done what you did. A year into our relationship you carried me into the hospital thinking I was dying. And then you stayed.

I didn't know your name but you taught me. I didn't know who you were, but you showed me. Above all this past year, you showed me what love is, and I thank you.

To the girls; from day one you all made it your mission to bring me home again. And you succeeded. I seriously can't imagine better friends. The laughs, the apple fights, the stroke rages, the late nights spent on the kitchen floor with the whiteboard explaining concepts to me, you've all been there every second. I freaking love you dudes.

To my team at Peterborough Regional Health Centre, I wouldn't be here without you. My neurologist, my doctors, the lab techs, the nurses, my speech pathologist, my outpatient physiotherapist, and the rest of the rehab team, thank you. K.B. and L.B., thank you for showing up every day. You gave me my life back and you allow me to live.

And finally, I thank myself. Thank you for taking the scary leap to write this book. For giving myself a piece of therapy I never knew how badly I needed. Thank you for continuing to live, to be yourself, and to navigate this world even with such doubt. I love you.

An Important Note About This Work

I wanted to give a few disclaimers before you read my story. First off, there is some minor swearing throughout this book. I recognize this may deter some readers. I tried to keep any inappropriate language to a minimum. However, there were some parts where I felt it was important to include the true language used to convey the seriousness of the situation, as well as to foster my true mental state during this time. Swearing was a part of my language use as I did not understand the difference between appropriate and inappropriate, and I had to re-develop a filter of speech.

When reading this book, you may come across spots that are not perfectly written. I am aware that this is the reality throughout this book. My editor/publisher, Lisa, and I have worked to make it flow nicely and be a good read. However, we also recognize the fact that I learned language skills less than a year ago (when writing this) and therefore it is not going to be perfect, nor should it. Please appreciate the value of the imperfection.

I also wanted to note that some names throughout this book have been changed to preserve confidentiality. All hospital staff names have been altered. However, most friends' and family members' true names are used as I received consent to include them.

A final note is that the timeline of these events is not definite. All events in this book are true to my life and did happen. I cannot, however, be sure of the exact order of the events. I tried to outline them as close to their exact date as I can remember, but it was a crazy time for all involved. So, if things are jumbled I apologize, but a lot happened fast. I promise that all things are true however. This is my story.

Chapter 1

I Should Probably Give Some Context

In December of 2021, I suffered a neurological episode that resembled a stroke. It severely changed my life. My stroke caused full left-side paralysis, left me unable to talk, and caused retrograde amnesia. It was like waking up as a foreigner in my own body and my own world. This book is the story of my experiences, the good and the bad, the happy and the messy, the successes and the breakdowns. It's my story of relearning the world from a fairly blank slate at the age of twenty-one. It is how I found myself in a world I know nothing about. How I refound my purpose and the reason I'm still here. This is my story and I hope you find some meaning in it as many others have said they have.

I wanted to note before we get deep into it that, as of yet, this neurological episode has not been diagnosed. There is unclear evidence of what happened. And in the wise words of my neurologist, we truly know so little about the brain and unless there is perfectly clear evidence about what happened, then we really aren't sure. Therefore I continue to be monitored, have regular scans done to keep an eye on the lesions, and otherwise just continue with my life as I want.

I have come to refer to my episode as a stroke as it makes the most sense to me. I was medically treated as a stroke patient as that was the closest connection at the time for my healthcare team. However, I want to be clear this is not a diagnosed stroke. But when you get a billion questions about what happened it is easier to say it's a stroke rather than an undiagnosed neurological episode that could be a stroke, MS, an autoimmune issue, or something else extremely rare. Therefore when not discussing my situation with new doctors, I choose to refer to it as a stroke so others (and I) understand what I mean. A stroke is how I will continue to refer to it in this writing.

* * *

When I sat down to start writing this, I truly had no direction, no idea how to do this or even what to write about. I didn't even register that people wrote books. The idea of how books came to be, had never occurred to me before. But I have been continuously told by many that I am an inspiration. Personally, I just see myself as a girl with some dreams, who isn't quite ready to let those dreams get pushed aside. However, since you are reading this, obviously I took people's advice and wrote about my experiences. I have decided that writing this truly serves one purpose for me; to be able to describe my experience in this crazy life. I really struggle to find words or to get people to understand what being in my mind is like. I really don't think it is possible to understand what it is like unless you have gone through something similar. So, I write to share my story, and as everyone likes to tell me, maybe I'll inspire someone else to keep going.

Before sharing my past crazy year, I wanted to start with a little back story about my life. I truly remember maybe 20% of my life before my stroke. So most of this recount is based on the lovely tellings of my family and friends.

I was born in Guelph, Ontario, and lived there for four years of my life. I then moved to Caesarea, Ontario, and continued to live there till my mid-teens. My mom, sibling and I moved to Port Perry when I was around 16, I believe. Then at 18, I moved to Peterborough to attend Trent University. Shortly after, in 2021, my mom moved to Bethany and I continued to split my time between her house and mine in Peterborough.

I believe I was a happy child, and did well in school, always active and on the go with different activities. A competitive dancer, an avid worker and just overall happy.

However, I went through my fair share of shit, it sounds like. I have always seemed to struggle medically. I was diagnosed with arthritis in my late teens as well as mast cell disorder. Apparently, in the two years leading up to my stroke, I basically lived at the hospital as they could not get my mast cell reactions under control. I was using as many epi pens a week as I could get my hands on, not by choice of course. As much as I don't have a recollection of these events, I have been told it was a real struggle. A struggle to stay in school, to work, to even just live a normal life. Almost dying every day sounds like it takes a toll on you.

Another thing I've come to find is that I have lost a lot of my family over the years. My uncle was arrested for pedophilia when I was a kid, and a lot of my family disapproved of my decision to not see, interact with, or support him. Therefore many of my relatives have lost contact with me from my mom's side.

My dad was in the picture until I was around 15 but I gather it was not a pretty picture with him either. I am grateful enough to not have all the memories of those times, but I still feel my sibling's pain. One Thanksgiving weekend, he woke up and he walked out on us. Jordan, my sibling, and I tried to restore a relationship with him of some form until it got too much to deal with. We stopped putting in effort and the contact between us dropped. My dad's whole side of my family never made an effort to stay connected with Jordan and me, as they see us as the problem in the situation. Therefore I have not spoken to anyone from my dad's side of the family in years and I wouldn't even be able to tell you who a single one of my paternal relatives are now.

I could tell you a lot more about the details of these situations. I could go on to tell you details about how people believe his lies about my mom keeping his kids from him, how my dad was an abusive narcissist, how my family says I'm disrespectful for not supporting my uncle, and the favourite line about forgiving and forgetting. But why would I waste time on that? Those people don't really deserve a mention, but I believed it was important to add some context to my life and to what my amazing family— Jordan, my mom and I — have already gone through.

So, on that note I want to mention the people that do matter. Except I decided to not mention them all right now, or else this introduction would turn into just a giant list of people's names! They will come up in the book as I write, and as they do, I hope they know that I am saying the most sincere *thank you* and *I love you*. I thank everyone, even those who don't know me but still support me. Thank you to those who care so deeply and love so much. Without you all this story wouldn't be possible.

So as I said, before my honourable mention tangent (just wait, there will be tons of those), I seemed to flourish in university. As I write this, I have graduated with my undergraduate degree in Psychology from Trent University. I completed it in April of 2022 (so, yes, after my stroke). And I am currently enrolled in two programs because I like to question my sanity every day. I am in a Master's of Science in Cognitive Psychology at Trent University, as well as doing an online postgraduate certificate in Human Resources Management from Fleming College.

As much as I joke about questioning my sanity, I am enrolled in two programs for a reason. School has proven to give me a purpose. When I had my stroke, school allowed me to prove to my medical team that I could keep going, and it gave me a drive. I need to have a fire under my ass, I need to have a driving force to keep me going. I am doing these two programs to get me where I want to go and to push me further toward my dreams. And those dreams are where I will get to.

But to get to my dreams, I have to tell my story, my struggle, and my path to creating myself. So let's get to all that good stuff.

Chapter 2

December 11, 2021

Pat and I are on our way home from having a nice date night out. A rare adventure for us as we navigate dating while being two of the busiest people alive. I always cherish the times we get to just be us. Be crazy, be wild, be in love, and be dumb together.

We went out for dinner as our time together has been quite limited lately while he was having his own life stuff happen. We went to a wing place in downtown Peterborough. If anyone knows the one I'm talking about, it all makes sense now why I ended up stroking out. Who actually goes to a dive bar for a rare date night?! Kidding... kind of...

So anyway, we had a nice night out. Ate some food, caught up and just enjoyed each other's company. As we head home I start thinking how nice of a night it was. Just us for once. I have felt good today. I had a headache on and off for the past few days but it had been a couple days since I had a mast cell reaction. I seem to be in an upcycle for the moment.

Pat pulls up to my place and I convince him to give me five more minutes of his precious time. We walk inside to find my roommates (often referred to as the girls) chatting and hanging out. They greet us in our front entryway. We all catch each other up about our days, and how Pat's and my date was. I move towards the stairs while talking. I sit down and begin to take my boots off. I place them on the shoe rack and continue to sit and chat.

Bright. It's bright. Colours, bright colours. Head hurts. Hurt.

Focus. You need to focus. Ignore the pain. Open your eyes, wait they are open. Focus. What is happening? Okay, there are people. Good, now who are those people, focus Jenna. Smile? Someone is asking you to smile. Okay now raise your arms? What? Pain. Pain. Pain. It's dark, I'm moving? I'm running, no I'm on a boat, no focus already. Black. Truck. "Get her in the truck." He's worried. His face is worried. Black.

Bright lights. God my head hurts.

"Are you fucking kidding me? I think she's having a stroke. Help her!" someone yells.

Blue. Blue fabric. Bright lights. Head hurts.

I'm sitting in a chair. Faces. Lots of faces. Where am I? A cute face. Who is that? He doesn't belong here, he isn't the same as the others. He isn't wearing the blue. He is different, I know him. Woah I can't feel that, that's a lot of needles in my arm. Why can't I feel it? Okay focus, they are asking you something. You need to answer. You need to figure out what happened, and where you are. Who are these people? They just moved me to a bed. They're taking my clothes off. Removing my nose ring? What the fuck. Bright lights. A tube? Where am I? Holy crap that burns. I'm peeing my pants, my skin is burning. My face is wet. Did I scream or is that in my head? How do I make it stop?

Wait it stopped. You need to focus.

Bright. I'm back to all the blue. They are all here again. Okay, a TV. Someone on the TV? Talking to me? That damn guy again is talking to this person. Who is he? Bright. My head still hurts. I need to close my eyes. He's arguing with the blue people.

Okay they've left me. It's just him. Who is he?

*My brain has left a gap here, I hypothesize it is a lot of the previous sequence on repeat.

A man in blue is here again.

He says, "The quick brown fox."

"Mmhmm."

What is that? Is that me talking? Oh god. I can't talk. I can't feel him touching my arm. Wait my leg. He's pricking me. Why can't I feel it? No not my face too. That guy is showing something with his face. Like pulling his face down. Bright. Blue. Bright. Pain in head.

Focus. What could this be? Where could I be?

Oh my gosh, no. No. No. I can't. No. That isn't right. That doesn't make sense. No.

I know this, I've studied this. But I can't do this. Bright, white, so bright. It hurts.

Calm down. Think of the facts. Okay, something is wrong with my talking, my head is killing me, the lights, the colours.

Colours.

Blue.

Focus. I can't feel my left side, but I can feel that guy holding my right hand. So one side is okay. The face pulling. Am I having a stroke? Oh my god, I am having a stroke. I can't die. I can't die. I. Cannot. Die.

Bright, it's so bright. It hurts, it hurts so bad. I'm gonna die. I'm done. Really this is how. I don't even know where I am and this is how I die.

Okay the blue people are back. Pull it together. Okay water, they have water. My mouth is dry. Drink. Oh god, I just dumped it down myself. The left side of my mouth is just dumping it out. This is bad. That damn guy is still here. How do I know him? Okay, the blue people left. He's gonna leave too he says. Where is he going? Wait. I reach out with my right hand and stop him.

I try to talk. "Uggg."

He tells me to stop, that it's okay, that my mom is here.

What does that mean? No, wait. I have to ask him something. It's there in my head. "Uggggg." *This is hard. He's trying to get it. I let go of his hand with my right hand. I start trying to use my hand to communicate.*

*I truly cannot recount how I communicated this next part.

But somehow I asked him if he was gonna leave me. He said yeah, my mom was here.

Mad. No, I mean forever, how doesn't he know this? How can he leave me? He is the only comfort I have right now.

Wait, he sees the frustration, he laughs. How can he laugh?

"Hun, that's what you're worried about right now? No I'm not going to leave you. Your mom is gonna come see you. I will be back." He leans down, kisses my head and is gone.

What did I even just ask him? I'm just so confused. Bright.

The pain is getting more tolerable.

A lady. I know her. But who is that? Wait he said my mom was here, whatever that means. Okay, well hi mom. The blue people talk to her. Oh god what are they doing to me now. Rolling me over, then back.

"Okay go pee."

Wait what? This man just told me to pee? My 'mom' and he are standing over me, watching me, talking to each other. Am I peeing? Just close your eyes.

*Another memory gap

Okay I'm in a hallway it looks like. Wait this must be a hospital. I've had a stroke. I'm in a hospital. Holy shit. How did this happen?

A man in blue leans over me. "Get up and walk." The 'mom' lady gets up, oh she's mad. They argue.

What are they saying? Why can't I hear them well? I can hear me, but not me, just my head me? This doesn't make sense. Stroke. That guy from before, I love him? 'Mom'? Who are these people? Bright. It still kinda hurts. The man in blue storms off. Mom tells me to sleep. Black. Hurts. Black.

*This all occurred between roughly 9 pm and 4 am. I was kept in the hospital hallway for a night before I got moved to a room in the emergency department as it was quite busy. There is a huge blank spot in my memory after this point until I was moved to the stroke floor. Probably because it consisted of the same thing, just waiting for a room and being given meds. I started to come to awareness a little more throughout these following days.

* * *

Pat walks into the room. He told me his name is Patrick. The people here refer to him as my boyfriend. He starts to show me all the gifts he brought from my 'roommates.' He pulls out this weird thing called a 'scone.' He starts to eat it. I refuse. The nausea is horrible. I can't eat. I am happy he gets to enjoy.

My eyes are heavy, but I feel happy when he is here. I'm scared.

He pulls something up on his phone. A game of some sort? He calls it football. Says we like to watch football. He watches the game. I pretend to watch it, but I watch him. Studying his face. Trying to remember.

My eyes are so heavy.

A lady comes in. Talks to us. I don't understand a lot of it. Says she is gonna ask me some questions. Starts showing me pictures.

That's a car.

I'm in one of those, that's a bed.

A pillow.

She asks me to say the things.

Why is this so hard to form these words? They are in my brain but won't come out.

She starts showing me physical objects.

A flashlight, they shine that in my eyes all the time.

What the hell are those? Oh god, what was that look between them? Obviously, I should know that then. Pat looks concerned. I have no idea what those are called, but I've seen them. (They are keys.)

The lady says to take a break and we will come back to it. She says she will see us later and leaves. We continue with the game on Pat's phone.

Sometime later, someone else comes into the room. A lady in those blue outfits. Says they have a room for me on the stroke floor.

The next hour of my life is a whirlwind. They move me to my room and immediately begin with testing. They prick my finger to get my blood (blood sugar testing). They swab different areas of my body. Draw a lot of blood. They collect my pee in a cup and then scan my bladder. They ask me about objects and once again I fail to name them.

Fuck. The worry is there, hiding in their faces.

A lady comes to do a physical assessment. My left side doesn't move, I can't feel it. I'm scared. There's a guy next to me in a bed. Talking to me. Saying how great I'm doing. Someone else brings in a wheelchair. Says she will be back to work with me tomorrow. So many questions asked of me, so many questions I have myself. Eventually, they all leave. Tell me to sleep because the same tests have to be done soon again. Pat makes sure I'm okay. Says he's gonna leave so I can sleep. Says my mom is coming again.

Sleep. Okay, I can sleep, my eyes are so heavy.

Sleep comes easy.

* * *

Upon recount, I've been told that the night of my stroke was not a great time. I have big patches missing from my memory of this night, and what I do remember took a while to come back to me.

My recount is somewhat correct, however. My boyfriend and I went out for dinner and then headed back to my place. I seemed fine to everyone around me. I was actively a part of the conversation when my roommates, Pat and I were all talking at my front entrance after dinner. I sat on the steps and took my shoes off. Then I just disengaged and slumped against the wall.

At first, my people thought I was having another allergic reaction as this was so common for me. But upon inspection, there was no swelling occurring. Rather my left side had gone basically dead. I had lost the ability to speak and my face was drooping. My one roommate called my mom and told her they weren't sure what was happening. Apparently, my mom tried to talk to me and there was no reaction from me.

Pat did in fact start asking me the typical stroke "FAST" questions. Got me to smile where one side didn't move and was drooped, my left arm wouldn't raise and I couldn't talk besides some weird groaning noises. My roommates threw my boots back on and they all got me out into Pat's truck. We live a quick 2-minute drive from the hospital so they decided he could have me there quicker than an ambulance could. So off we went.

When we got there, the obscured treatment began. Pat carried me in and immediately took me to the closest nurse. As this was during the pandemic, there were screeners at the door who argued with Pat about me not wearing a mask and not sanitizing my hands. I correctly remember him saying something along the lines of "Are you fucking kidding me?" in response.

After having a mask slapped on my face, he was able to bring me to the triage desk. They got me into a wheelchair, did a quick intake and rushed me to the back. Pat recalls all available staff jumping on me. Blood sugar testing (normal), pupil testing (one pupil was dilated, the other wasn't), IV inserted, scratch testing on the two sides of my body for feeling, and every other test they could do in that time. The ER doctor remembered me from being there the other day with an allergic reaction.

Due to this, the two ER doctors that handled me that night quickly became unprofessional. They came up with the idea that I was faking it as I had been in the emergency room often with anaphylaxis. I would like to note that there is well-documented evidence that my anaphylactic reactions from my mast cell disorder are real. I have pictures, numerous ambulance rides and hospital stays documented, and lots of reports of doctors having to give me secondary shots of epinephrine as they watched my throat close in the hospital. I truly don't see the joy I would get out of using epi-pens, nor would the doctors just give me multiple rounds of epi if they didn't think I needed it.

However, the two doctors on shift on December 11, 2021, had a different idea. Immediately they believed I was faking my paralysis and such. They made claims such as seeing my foot move, even though Pat was watching it and saw nothing. Nor did the nurses see anything. The doctors waited a while before doing an emergency CT scan. It wasn't until, as they stated, they "had no choice" but to do one because I wasn't improving. So reluctantly, they put me through a CT. In their words, it came back relatively normal (Pat questioned what that meant and got no explanation.) They then consulted with a neurologist from Toronto who said she was unsure what was happening but believed I needed an MRI as soon as possible, and that I should not be released at least until I got one.

The doctors did not follow this recommendation. They said they were gonna give me a bit to see if my symptoms improved. I believe they did start me on blood thinners at this point but then left me alone.

At this point, Pat and my mom switched out. Eventually, I was moved to the hallway as my room was needed by someone else. I lay in the hallway for hours with my mom, who tried to get me to sleep. Around 3:00 am, the one ER doctor finally came back to check on me.

As my mom recounts, he told me to get up and walk. My mom refused to even let me try and asked how the hell I was going to do that, all while I just stared at him. His response was, “Well I guess we will have to admit her then if she refuses to walk.” My mom said something like, “Yes, you will admit her so we can figure out what’s wrong.” The doctor made a snide comment to my mom about me faking it and how it’s the same as my ‘fake’ anaphylactic reactions. And then he walked away. We remained in the hallway alone.

Eventually, they did move me to a room within the ER. After shift change the next morning, the new nurse did an assessment and couldn’t believe our story. She reassured me that there was no way I was faking it. She also informed us that the ER doctor had not in fact started the admitting or MRI process but rather just left me. We had to wait until the next doctor started their shift for them to assess me and start the admitting process. I remained in the ER for about 3 days, I believe, before they had a bed for me on the stroke floor. And the treatment became a miracle once I was moved there.

I would like to just take a moment for myself and state that if those two ER doctors ever hear of my story, I truly hope they can reflect on their choices and never put someone else through this. Not only for me but for others in my situation. My mom heard one of them yell at a patient to “pay attention already” after they were diagnosed with a stroke. So obviously the poor lady was confused, but the doctor still yelled at her.

The cruel treatment really sets the tone for any issue, regardless of the severity. And I wish more people recognized this. Whether I was having a stroke or not, I deserved respect. If I was faking it, why send me home? Obviously, my mental health is not okay if I were to fake a stroke. So where is the psychiatry consult, the social work support, the compassion because something is going on? No, rather, 'Get up and walk and get out' was the treatment given. So if you are like these doctors or, even better, if you do happen to be these two men, then I encourage you to reflect on your actions. And either change your behaviour or change your career. Because you don't deserve to be there to treat others how you treated me. One night turned into 49 days in the hospital and a lifetime of recovery. And how you treated me will never leave me. I hope one day to have the opportunity to hear your honest apology. But that is a big hope in my small world.

Chapter 3

December 14, 2021

Bree comes into my room. My second time meeting her. She was the one who dropped me off a wheelchair the previous night. She writes her name on my board. Bree, I like that name. *She looks kind.*

She and Pat run through my story of how I ended up here. It feels like the billionth time I've heard this; I think I've memorized what has happened because of every single person asking. Once they are done getting through the events leading up to this moment, Bree asks me if anyone has gotten me out of bed yet. I tell her the nurses have only gotten me up for the numerous tests they ran this morning, consisting of a head MRI, spine MRI and an EEG. She explains that with the wheelchair I can have more freedom to roam the floor on my own, and I tell her I would like that. That is all it took for our work to begin.

Bree grabs the wheelchair, brings it to my bedside and says "Let's do this!" I raise my bed up to a sitting position. We place a pillow under my left arm to support it in the transfer. Bree instructs me to use my good arm to gently swing my left leg off the side of the bed. I do so and then swing my right leg over the same side so I'm sitting up on the side of the bed.

From here we do a few assessments of balance. I'm instructed to hold myself upright as best as possible as Bree gently pushes me sideways. My left ab muscles don't engage and I immediately flop over onto my side. My right side holds up fine thanks to Mom and me doing all those ab workouts pre-stroke.

Once Bree assesses where I am at, it is time to get me into my wheelchair. She teaches me how to do a pivot turn into the chair off the side of my bed. The rehab team in my room supports my left side, while I use my right leg to stand and pivot into my chair. It's a little rocky the first few attempts but eventually we get there.

Even just moving to my chair is exhausting but it feel so good to have that small amount of mobility. In my exhausted state, I assume that is enough for one day and that I can pivot back to bed and be done. But I quickly realize that I will not be off the hook that easily. Bree tells me I did great and that it is time to head to the gym.

The previous day, I saw other people on the floor move their wheelchairs using one hand and one foot. So I pick up the technique quickly and follow Bree to the gym.

When we get to the gym, it is quite overwhelming. I don't know what half the things in here are. But the rehab team present is quick to greet me with kindness and assurance. Bree pushes me over to a set of bars in front of a mirror. She asks some of the other rehab team members to come over and help out. They strap a support belt around my waist and tell me I'm going to stand.

I start to freak out about how I can do that. I have one freaking leg. But they quickly reassure me that I will be okay. They remind me that three staff are there helping me, and weight-bearing through my left leg is the best way to start to get the blood flowing through it, and possibly some feeling back.

So I take a breath and tell myself I can do it. They tell me to try and stand to see where I'm at and my technique. I take a big breath and push as hard as I can upwards with my right leg. I don't even get my butt an inch off the chair. It seems impossible. However, I receive encouragement all around for trying.

A physiotherapist, Trish, then tells me that there is a technique to it. She first gets me to 'butt scooch' to the edge of the seat, using my right arm to push my left side forward. Once I'm sitting close to the edge I place my right leg at a 90-degree angle with the floor, and Bree holds my left leg in place. Trish gets me to place my right hand on the bar in front of me and another team member holds my left hand beside it on the bar. She instructs me to lean forward and then try pushing up like a squat. With a lot of struggle, a lot of Trish and Bree lifting on my support belt, and a lot of encouragement from Pat, I stand up.

I get this wild feeling of blood rushing through my body. It's the first time standing in days and it feels so weird. 'Whoop whoop!" The room breaks out into cheers for me. And then the rehab team helps me sit. I'm exhausted. My head is starting to hurt more and my right side feels like I did an intense workout. Bree tells me to call it a day as that was amazing and that we can try to stand again tomorrow.

While being pushed back to my room, I begin thinking. *Are you kidding me? I stood up. I stood up once, for ten seconds. And I'm exhausted. And you all say that's amazing. You all are walking around like nothing, pushing me back to my room, and you think I just did a good job by having someone haul my ass out of a chair. That's bullshit. Is this my new life?*

Even with my angry, swirling thoughts, I'm too tired to do or say anything. With a lot of help, I complete another pivot transfer back into my bed from my wheelchair. I try to stay awake and talk to Pat but my eyelids slide closed.

But not for long.

"Hi Jenna, do you remember me?"

I turn towards the voice, I know that face.

"It's Kara; I work here as a speech therapist. I saw your file come across my desk and had to come to see you. You used to volunteer at my work with the aphasia group."

Holy shit, I do know this person. Why don't I know anyone else? But I know her.

Kara continues, "I'm really sorry we had to meet this way again. But I'm glad to see you. This may be weird but I wanted to ask if you are okay with me working with you. If you aren't comfortable with it, that is totally okay, someone else can take on your case."

I grin and nod. In choppy speech I get out "I, I, I, I, would loooo-love for you to wwwww-work with me. It's like having a friend here, sssss-someone I know."

"Aww, that's great, I will let you rest but I will come back tomorrow to start some speech therapy with you."

Pat turns to me and asks, "How do you know her?" It takes me a while but eventually together I work out the story that I used to volunteer at an aphasia group in Peterborough. She ran the program and I volunteered as a communication assistant for a few years. I hadn't seen her since I couldn't volunteer anymore at the start of the pandemic.

This moment is a glimmer of hope. Maybe there are still things in my brain. Maybe some memories are still in there, I just have to find them.

Pat decides it is time for him to head out, and it is time for me to sleep. The nurse comes in and does the cognitive testing that I have to get every 4 hours. I still can't figure out what that one object (keys) is but otherwise, I do alright. My blood sugar is good, my bladder is emptying properly and my pupil has gone back to normal. Sleep comes easy after my tests are done.

****

I have a roommate here in the hospital. His name is Paul. He has suffered a serious stroke and a heart attack due to the stroke. He also has paralysis as well as short-term memory loss. In the brief time I've been here, Paul has been an amazing companion; he constantly reminds me how brave and strong I am and his intuition about my feelings is crazy.

The nurses have just dropped our breakfast off to us. I look at my plate and read the paper with the menu, trying to relearn what this food is. One of the items is a banana. I quickly grab my phone and search up bananas. I see that you peel them and enjoy the fruit inside.

I pick up my banana and study it for a minute. I then try to peel it as I saw on my phone. I can't get it. I lay the banana on my food tray and try to peel the top with my right hand. It just keeps sliding across the tray. I begin to feel extremely frustrated. I don't even know what this food is and now I can't even eat it properly.

Tears start to well up in my eyes.

"Hey Jenna," Paul says.

"Ya," I reply.

"Do you need help with your breakfast? I remember having to learn how to peel these silly bananas. I'll call the nurse for us. I struggle too," Paul says.

I almost start laughing. How does he know I'm struggling? The curtain between our beds is closed, he can't even see me.

I realize Paul gets it. He's been here and now he can support me. In the past few days, he has already become a motivation for me. Knowing he has been here for months already makes me want to work as hard as him.

His smile, his determination, and his kindness are infectious. His wife has even been cheering me on since we met the other day. Our bond will keep growing stronger. An odd pair of a 60-year-old man and a 21-year-old gal in their separate hospital beds, but a pair with a strong never forgotten bond.

****

It is dinnertime and I am quickly beginning to realize that hospital food is not where it is at. As I eat I begin to feel sad and alone. It is scary not knowing anyone, not knowing what has happened.

Paul starts to talk to me; he seems to always sense when I need a friend. He tells me about his family, his grandkids, and he even shows me pictures. He tells tales of his time as a firefighter. And I soak it all up. As Paul and I are talking, someone walks into the room. Surprisingly they aren't wearing the blue scrubs I have gotten used to. Wait, this face seems familiar. I smile; their smile is infectious.

It turns out to be my roommate from home and one of my closest friends, Bella. It is a glorious sight to see her. It takes me a bit to connect the dots about who she is, but the familiar feelings of *her* are there. She has brought me a blanket and a few things from home. As much as I don't remember the things she has brought me, they feel comforting because I know they are mine from home. She even brought me her 'house cardigan' to wear as a comfort item from all my friends. I love it, it makes me feel a little bit more like I will be okay, like I am safe and protected.

We go through each thing she brought me. She explains them all to me. As we finish, I ask her to keep talking, I like it. She updates me about all the things happening at home. All the stuff my friends are doing, who my friends even are, and all the new tea in their lives (as the youth like to say). Bella has this sense about me even from prior when I was sick with my mast cell disorder, she always knows when I'm drained but fighting it.

"Wanna get ready for bed? I can stay and talk or even watch something but let's get the hard part done with," Bella says.

I quickly reject her help. I point to my call bell and work out "I will get the nurses to help me."

"Dude I love you, I've worked in care homes all my life, changing you will be nice, you're young and not all wrinkled," Bella says while laughing.

I quickly come to gather that arguing with Bella is not going to work, so reluctantly I let her pick out pyjamas for me. I internally feel so vulnerable, so weak, alone, raw. Here I am sitting in a bed, half paralyzed, letting my friend change me. A week ago I was dancing at a bar, writing my thesis, and doing whatever my heart wanted, and yet here I sit unable to do anything for myself.

Bella gets my pyjamas and changes me. I need to start to learn how to do more of this myself. That is one of my next goals.

Once my pyjamas are on, Bella helps me slide over to the side of my bed. She comes onto the bed and lies beside me. She grabs my laptop and gets a movie started. I lay my head on her shoulder and doze off with my rediscovered friend.

Upon reflection, this is the start of my struggle with my new self. The truth of my symptoms, my condition, it sets in and it becomes a rocky road. In my opinion I handled this situation with as much realistic positivity as possible. I had great moments of defeat, but overall not once did I turn down a rehab session, not once did I give up, and not once did I choose to stop fighting. The people around me, hospital staff and family, handled it beautifully. Bella dealt with this situation (plus many others) with such grace; it was unbelievably comforting. When I went on to scream at a nurse for trying to talk to me as she held me on the toilet, she accepted my anger and apologized. I was not her typical clientele (as in I was below the age of 60) and she forgot how odd this must all be for me. When I sat naked in a shower room crying, with two nurses washing me for the first time, they made sure to braid my hair after and silently comfort me because words were too much. Those who I grew to call my people accepted my raw emotions, my vulnerability, my anger that was unjustly thrown at them, and my many, many tears. It was all accepted with love. It allowed me to grieve the *me* I'd lost, to start my journey of growth, of healing, of creating this new self in this strange world.

It took about three days after my stroke for my grief to set in, and it seems like it will take a lifetime to heal, but my god I wouldn't change this journey for the world.

Chapter 4

December 16, 2021

I hold up my paper for them to read. My face is firm, I've made my decision. "I don't care, I'm writing it," I say.

"Jenna, we are worried about this. Not that we don't think you can do it, but it's stress you don't need. Your brain needs to heal, it doesn't need this. We know you can do it, you don't have to prove it to us. We know you're capable. Take the break. It could be too much, I don't want to see this crush you or make you too tired. You're capable Jenna but it is a lot for you right now," Sarah, my speech pathologist, says.

"I keep telling her, she is pushing too hard," my nurse, Ryan, chimes in.

"No," I firmly say. I've come to like this word, I can get it out easy and it's firm; it's quickly becoming a favourite, as Jordan would say.

"Okay, then we have a lot of work to do. I'll get Kara to start researching psychology terms and maybe Bree can do some testing with you," Sarah says reluctantly.

"Yup, I'm on it! I'll come to get you for the gym later and we can write a test or something down there," Bree says with an encouraging tone.

"Okay, and are you okay if Bree and I also meet with your professor? I know you and Pat met with her but maybe we should check in as well just so she knows the scope of the situation," Sarah asks.

"Okay," I reply.

Sarah leaves but Bree sticks around. "I get why you're doing this. I'm gonna work with you; we are gonna make this happen."

"Thank you," I reply.

And off she goes till later. I have one final exam to write for this semester and I want to write it. I could easily be given an option to not write it, but I am refusing that. I want to prove I can do something for myself and for everyone else. My speech and language pathologist has tried to talk me out of it, along with many of my nurses. They aren't rude about it, and I get where they are coming from; it probably isn't good for me to do, but I need to do something. In rehab, I've been able to stand and do some squats. I'm starting to get tingling in my left side which they say is a really good sign, I just think it's annoying. My speech is also making progress but each day we are finding more and more things that I can't name or say. I have begun to be able to talk again in sentences which is nice but I have a moderate level stutter. As well, I'm suffering from aphasia. I struggle to understand speech sometimes, words get trapped in my head and won't come out, and sometimes I say the wrong word while I am thinking I am saying something else. It's become an ongoing joke to see how many times I say cup in a day. I call everything a cup without meaning to. My support team and I even say 'I cup you' instead of I love you.

It almost feels like each day I have a win that feels so good, such as my finger flinches, or I move my toe a centimetre, but then I step back and think about how little that win is. It's defeating.

So this exam is a chance to do something, to not sit back and take the easy way out and not write it. Are my nurses right and I'm working myself too hard? Yes, but that isn't new, I've been told. That's the Jenna my family has always known. So, much to everyone's dismay, I refuse to take a pass on this exam. I refuse to not take courses next semester, I refuse to give up on school. I have two courses and my thesis left to finish before I graduate. I am in the process of finishing up my grad school applications. Why the hell would I stop here?

It's nice to have Bree on my side. My family is also supportive; they think I'm crazy but they are supportive nonetheless. Pat and I met with my professor over zoom and explained the situation. She has been super supportive and accommodating. She's giving me up until the last minute to decide if I want to write it or not. But we all know I will write it.

Sarah and Bree want to talk to her. I know their worry is from a good place, but it still annoys me. I love my rehab team here; they are so encouraging and push me to keep going. But they also know when

I should stop, even if I don't. I just hope their meeting goes well enough with my professor that we all agree to let me write the exam.

I sit alone with my thoughts for a bit and take a little snooze. Soon afterwards, my mom shows up.

She has been coming a lot, which is nice, but I also feel guilty. She says she doesn't mind; however, I can't imagine how hard it is for her to balance work, supporting Jordan, and me being in the hospital.

But every day she comes to see me, helps me pivot to my wheelchair, and we go together and get a coffee downstairs at the coffee shop. It's become a little tradition that I've learned to love. I think she enjoys it too. We often go up to the top floor of the hospital; we call it 'our spot.' There is a window corner where I can overlook part of the city and almost imagine myself out there. Imagine myself running through the streets, the forests, hearing the birds that sit on the window ledge, hear the ambulances drive by, listen to the kids laugh at the nearby park, and explore those stores out there. There is so much for me to experience, and this window spot is as close as I'll get to that for a while. After we spend time drinking our coffee and watching the world at our spot, my mom will push me around the hallways.

After the first week, this novelty has lost some of its excitement. There is not as much to look at as you think there is in a hospital. However, besides our spot, I do particularly enjoy the 'whiteboard of dreams,' as I call it. It is a whiteboard located near the I.T. section of the hospital, on the upper floors. It often has a question on it and then many people's responses. My mom and I have made it part of our adventures to go and check it out regularly. It is almost like having friends in this place.

Other than our whiteboard of dreams, the only other really exciting thing to look at is the artwork on the bottom floor. It's the psych floor and they have this weird connected set of art. It is a bunch of canvases painted solid colours, that are displayed down the hallways and they range from blues to purples to greens to reds and all the colours in between. It seems like weird art to me, but it has allowed me to learn my colours easily. I've gone to look at these numerous times and each time they get easier to name but the concept is just as weird to me. However, we still go and look.

After a while of roaming the hallways, I tend to get exhausted so we head back to my room. Once we are there, we either curl up in my bed, throw on a movie and I sleep, or if my brain can handle it then we do some rehab work.

On this particular day, my mom came earlier in the day, so we take our coffee and walk around lunchtime. We head back to my room with enough time for me to have a little rest before my afternoon rehab. As much as you are supposed to rest in the hospital, there really isn't that much time for it. Nights are loud with alarms, call bells and the typical check-ins. My days are jam-packed with as much rehab as I can fit in, so any chance I can get to rest, I take it.

Just as I start to doze off, there is a knock at my door and Bree comes in.

"Wanna hit the gym before speech?"

"Yes," I say with a smile.

Bree comes to my bed and helps me to pivot myself into my wheelchair. Off we roll to the gym.

When we get there, I start with a warm-up on the bike. We strap my left foot in and then I pedal with my right foot. Most of the work is being done by my right but the movement does bring pins and needles to my left leg. After doing this for five minutes, Bree stops the bike. We move over to the bench and start with some arm exercises. At this point they are pretty basic, just working on getting my fingers to wiggle.

"Have you been doing the weight-bearing exercises?" Bree asks.

"Yeah, I try to do them a few times each night before bed."

"They seem to be a little better; you need less elbow support," chimes in my mom.

"Good, it will get there. Alright, today let's switch it up a little from our squats and weight bearing. Roll on over to the parallel bars," Bree says.

I roll up in between the bars. Bree grabs a stool and goes through to the other side of them so we are facing each other. My mom of course gets out her phone to film the session.

Bree says we are going to start with some weight shifting as we've done before.

I stand out of my chair and place my left hand on the left bar and grab the right bar with my right hand. Bree holds my hips and I shift my weight back and forth. The left side is unsteady but I keep trying to put weight onto it. Bree and the rehab assistants support my left hip and knee as I put weight into them, so they don't collapse.

Bree then instructs me to try and lift my feet off the ground as I weight shift. My eyes grow twice the size and I begin to panic.

"Relax, I'm here, we've got you. Just take it slow and try. You have the bars, you have the three of us staff. You can do it."

I take a big breath and tell myself I can do it. I shift to the right and awkwardly lean really far over to make my left leg come off the ground.

"Good, now try the other side," Bree encourages.

So I lean to the left, my right hand death-gripping onto the bar, and I slowly take my right foot about an inch off the ground. Instantly pins and needles shoot down my left leg and my knee starts to collapse. I plant my right foot on the ground again and a rehab assistant brings my wheelchair up behind me so I can sit.

"That was so good! What did it feel like?" exclaims Bree.

"Weird, and scary. It gave me pins and needles in my leg," I explain.

"That's a good sign, as annoying as it is. It means the nerves are starting to wake up again in your leg," says Trish, the physiotherapist.

I explain where exactly I felt them in my leg and rate them on the pain scale. We talk about it for a few minutes and then Bree says, "Alright let's go again."

So up I stand and we do it a few more times. Once I'm breathless and my leg won't hold me anymore, we end the session.

"I'll give you the rest of the afternoon off because you still have speech work to do, but keep weight bearing a bit tonight when your nurses take you to the bathroom. Take a moment to put some weight into that leg. I'll see you tomorrow!" Bree says.

"Thank you guys, that was great!" I reply.

My mom and I roll back to my room to wait for my speech session.

"I'm so proud of you Jen, you're doing so well," my mom says.

"Thank you, I'm trying," I reply.

When we get back to my room we just start to rest for a few minutes until it's speech time.

Kara comes to grab me, I roll down to the speech room and we start. Today is warming up with some basic object recognition. Kara pulls objects out of a box and I have to name them and their function. We start with the normal ones I get asked every morning and night for my neuro-checks.

"Flashlight for seeing things, pen to write, watch to tell time, cup," I say.

"Good but try again," Kara says.

"Cup, cup, cup."

"Let's do it together. Gl-ass-es," Kara says slowly.

"Gl-ass-ssss."

"Good! That was really good Jenna!" Kara exclaims.

We continue with our naming for a bit longer while I also practice my new strategies of mouth-watching and mimicking, writing stuff down, taking things slow, and using my alphabet board.

After naming objects is done, we switch to just doing some talking exercises. Kara asks me simple questions such as how is your day going, and what did you have for lunch? I talk for a bit, working through my stutter. Then we go on to discuss my psychology course. Kara explains that she is going to start to do some work in our speech lessons with psychology terms. I show her my notes and activities from class and we decide on key things I should study. By the end of it, I am exhausted.

"You did great today. Go take a rest, that was a lot," Kara says.

"I'm so proud of you Jenna," my mom says.

"Thank you," I reply, and start wheeling myself back to my room.

Just as I get back to my room, Bree pokes her head in, "Hey, tomorrow morning when we go to the gym I'm going to give you a psychology quiz that I made up from online using development questions for your exam. Be prepared! And then in the afternoon, we will try some more arm work."

"Oh great! Can't wait," I reply and off she goes.

"That will be good!" my mom says. "But now rest; take a little nap before dinner. Are you okay if I go? There is going to be a surprise for you tonight."

"What is that?" I ask.

"Someone is going to come and see you, but I am not going to tell you who. You have to wait and see."

"Okay fine," I say, too tired to question it further.

My mom packs up her stuff and heads out, and I close my eyes.

* * *

"Hey kid!" In walks Jordan just as I finish my dinner. I know this person! I know who Jordan is! I am so freaking excited to finally know someone; it's a relief that I'm not completely lost.

My face lights up as they sit at the end of my bed. "Hhhi!" I say excitedly.

"You excited to see me?" Jordan asks.

"Yes!" I say.

"Good! It's nice to see you. I brought you some surprises," Jordan says.

Just as they start to unpack their bag of goodies, a nurse comes in. "A new visitor! Who is this?" they ask.

"My sibling, Jordan," I say.

"Well it's nice to meet you Jordan. I just need a few minutes to do a neuro check before I shift change and then I will leave you two to hang," the nurse says.

I go through the process of a neuro check and then turn my attention back to Jordan. I explain to them through talking and writing on my new speech notepad that now we have time before I have to do my next neuro check so we can explore a bit. I'm excited to show off my new home as well as my wheelchair skills. Jordan finishes showing me everything they* packed for me, including clothes, some personal hygiene items and a surprise of their stuffed monkey, Chester, who is my new roomie until I get to go home. I thank them and they help me put away my stuff into the cupboard by my bed.

With Jordan's help, I transfer to my wheelchair and off we go to begin our tour. I show them the nurses' station, the gym, the speech room and the showers on the floor. Then Jordan offers to take me around the hospital for a little roll before bed, and I gladly agree. We tour the hospital, and I show Jordan all my favourite spots.

"Let's go to Tims, kid. I could use a tea and you're working hard. This calls for doughnuts!" Jordan says. When we get there, I ask Jordan to pick me out something as I am unsure of what to get. Jordan orders themselves a tea and two chocolate doughnuts.

"This is my favourite kind of donut. You used to like it but if you don't then I get two!" Jordan jokes with me.

We roll back to my room and Jordan gives me my doughnut. I take a bite and think *damn this is so good compared to the food I've been given.* I give Jordan a smile and thumbs up.

* Jordan identifies as non-binary, and is referred to as they/them in this book.

"I'll take it you like it kid!" Jordan says.

I nod happily.

We eat our snack while Jordan goes on about their days lately and I listen intently. I try to soak up all the information everyone else says, they all seem to know so much. I want to know it all too.

Jordan talks about their day, their work, our friends who I don't remember. They ask me questions about knowing things and mostly I shake my head no and then they explain. Jordan also asks me questions to relay the information back to them. I become frustrated as it's like my whole life with everyone has become one big rehab and therapy work session, but I try not to get frustrated at my people. I don't want them to stop visiting. Plus it seems to make them happy so I try my best to go along with it.

Jordan explains what they do for work and tells me a story about one of their clients. Then they stop and ask, "So what do I do for work?"

"You do the homeless," I say.

Jordan starts laughing. "Not exactly, kid, but close enough." Jordan keeps laughing. I'm confused at what is so funny but I laugh along because it seems like the thing to do. (Jordan does not in fact 'do the homeless'; they are a housing first caseworker for a non-profit housing organization, but I was close.)

Jordan continues to talk with me for a bit longer, until they see me getting tired. They help me wheel to the bathroom, and brush my teeth. Then I call the nurse, who helps me use the bathroom, changes me into PJs, gives me meds, does a neuro check, and then helps me into bed. Jordan tucks me into my bed after the nurse leaves.

"I love you kid, hang in there; you'll be home soon," Jordan says as they get ready to leave.

"I love you too Jordy," I work out in broken speech.

"Jordy, you remember that eh?" Jordan says with a smile.

I smile and nod; they kiss my head and walk out. I let my heavy eyes close and drift away for the night.

Chapter 5

December 21, 2021

The days are a flurry of daily routines. Wake up with rounds by 7, do my neuro tests, and meds, then have breakfast.

The nurses always come in and help me get ready after breakfast. I've had my first few showers, which has been humiliating for me but well-needed. The nurses always ensure that I am doing alright. They even often take the time to braid my hair out of my face as I am still getting used to not being able to tie it up with only one hand.

After the nurses get me ready, it's rehab time. Physiotherapy followed by occupational therapy.

Lunch break and rest.

Then more rehab; physio, OT and speech.

Then dinner break and rest.

The days finish with visiting time and more speech/neuro work with my visitors.

The days are exhausting but fly by quickly. I have gotten my bearings about what has happened. I finally feel comfortable in this setting. The hospital feels like home to me.

I have, however, switched rooms. The nurses told me it was more appropriate to be in my own room given my age and all the other patients' ages on the floor. As well, being a young girl who needs help with everything, it was more appropriate to not be placed with an older gentleman in the same situation. Therefore the nurses moved me to a private room. I still go to visit my old roommate Paul, bring him coffee when I get one, and we chat in the gym. But I am now in my own room.

I am starting to get minor feeling back in my left side. The feeling in my face is back completely, and the droop had subsided. As well I get less intense headaches and can do therapy for a little longer each day. Still not long, but for some sessions (the morning ones when I was fresh to the day) I can last almost 20 minutes in the gym! I can even slowly wiggle some of my fingers and toes. It is so exciting for all of us.

I am beginning to appreciate the small wins. A wiggle in one finger was more than I had the day before, and the excitement from my support and rehab team makes me excited about it as well.

My neuro checks have also been reduced to only morning and night instead of every four hours, which is nice. I can now sleep through the night without being woken up to check my pupils, blood sugar, do an object recognition task and all the other fun things.

I enjoy the routine and the hard work that is involved here. It makes my days better.

I also have learned to love the evenings. I am lucky enough to have a huge circle of people who want to see me, so I am never alone. In addition to my evening visits, I am always on a video call with someone during my early breakfast and lunch breaks. Due to Covid-19 the hospital policy is that I am only allowed one visitor at a time but it can be whoever I want.

Therefore, I let my mom handle the fights about who is coming to visit me. And I fit people into my video call schedule.

Within the first two weeks of being here in the hospital I have already seen so many of my people. My roommate Julia has visited a few times, my friend Connor has come, my brother Logan took me to Tim Hortons inside the hospital for dinner, and took me outside for the first time to experience the air, I had an experience of re-trying ice cream with Bella my roommate, my brother Andrew brought me my first McDonalds meal, and I had many visits with my mom and Pat. My mom also came up with a brilliant plan of doing outside visits. She comes in the evenings and wheels me outside so many people can see me at once. I have had visits with my family, friends and roommates.

Even the people I call my bonus family came to see me. My bonus family includes; my favourite little kiddo Addie, my second set of parents Leisa and Cameron, or as I like to call them 'Mom and BBQ Dad,' and their other kids, Amy and Eric. Even their dog came to see me. I had wheelchair races with Addie and relearned all their names.

(But just like I had with Jordan, I always remembered who Addie was. Those are the two people I never forgot.)

It is so nice to know I am so loved by all these people coming to visit.

Through these visits, we have learned something unique about my memory loss. As we've noticed, I don't remember who people are. I've had to be reintroduced to all my friends and family, except for Jordan and Addie.

However, for those I do not remember, it turns out I remember facts about them without realizing it. When I see people, sometimes a thought jumps into my head and I yell it out loud. I have no idea where these thoughts come from or what they mean. But they are actually related to the person. So their name is not known in my mind but things about them are in my unconscious memory.

For example, when I refer to Cameron from my bonus family as BBQ Dad, it is because I yelled out BBQ Dad when I saw him for the first time the other day. I had no idea what this meant but my mom and Leisa immediately started laughing. Prior to my stroke, I always thought of him like a dad, especially when I lived with them for a while during the prior lockdowns. And if you are ever looking for Cameron, just find the nearest barbeque and there he will be with a beer in his hand at his happy place. Hence me calling him BBQ Dad meant I remember him, it's just trapped somewhere inaccessible in my brain.

Cameron is not the only instance of this, however. I always call Pat 'cute guy,' but maybe that is just because I think he is pretty cute. I call Ellen 'coffee whore' as she used to drink buckets of coffee a day. My brother Andrew is named 'Andy Cowboy' to me as he came to my Halloween party dressed as a cowboy this past year (I'll spare you from your other nickname, Andrew, you can thank me later!). My friends Jackie and Tara are coined 'Chuck Chuck and Jack Jack' and 'Baseball' because Tara is a baseball player. There are many other nicknames I have created to remember people, but you get the gist. I find it interesting to know that these memories of people are still somewhere in my mind, I just have to find them.

These new learnings that have been occurring the past few days are interesting and keeping me going. It gives me a reason to fight through the emotions, the pain, the grief. It allows me to believe that I may be able to recover all my memories, that I may walk again one day, that I may return to school, and may achieve all my dreams.

So each day, I take it one minute at a time and just try my best to learn everything I can, soak up all the knowledge and information possible and work as hard as ever to make my rehab goals a reality. I am beginning to appreciate this life and be happy with the new me, regardless of my new limits.

* * *

Bree walks into my room and says, "I've got some bad news."

I sit up in bed and look at her, feeling worried.

"So there is an announcement coming down later today and I wanted you to know about it. I'm going to let you know what is happening as soon as I know, but there are going to be some changes. We are going into another lockdown and therefore stronger Covid restrictions. I know Julia is supposed to come tomorrow to assist you with communicating in your exam but you might not be allowed any visitors after today. It's rumoured there are going to be no visitors but I'm going to fight for you," she says.

I feel upset but I nod my head in understanding.

"Also there's more, I'm sorry. Like I told you earlier this week, you're on the list for a Christmas day pass. It got approved this morning for you to go for the day. But with these new restrictions coming down, we aren't sure if anyone will be allowed to go home. You might not get your day pass. I'm sorry. I swear I'm going to try everything for you," Bree says sadly.

"I'm upset," I respond, "but it isn't your fault. Can we just go to the gym? I don't want to think about this right now."

"Yup! Let's go," Bree says as she spots me to do a pivot turn into my wheelchair.

We head to the gym as I work on distracting myself from the visitor news. We do some light rehab work. Bree doesn't want to push me too hard because she wants me to be rested for my exam tomorrow. We do some work on the arm and leg bike, some weight shifting and some arm weight bearing. We are having a lot of trouble getting any movement in my arm and we cannot figure out why. But every day we try our best to get it moving as much as we can.

After finishing up our session, Bree tells me I am good to head back to my room. "Hey Jenna, before you go. I just want you to know, I think you'll be ready to try some steps soon. Just so you're prepared," Bree says with a big smile.

"Really?!" I replied, half super excited, half wanting to faint with nerves.

"Yup, it's your next goal. I'll see you tomorrow afternoon. Take this afternoon to rest and study. But once your exam is over we are going hard with rehab. Get a good sleep tonight, you've got this. I'll come to wish you luck before you start in the morning."

"Thanks Bree," I say as I roll back to my room.

Wow, steps, I think to myself. Am I really ready? Well if Bree thinks so then yeah, she knows me better than I do. I just have to get through tomorrow morning and then it's walking time!

I take out my school notes once I'm back in my room and start studying while trying to push the idea of walking out of my head.

* * *

"Hey. I'm just about to head out but I wanted to check in. How is studying?" Bree asks.

"Good. I feel good, but tired," I reply.

"Make sure you get good sleep tonight. It's gonna be a tough day for you. But you've got it," Bree says.

"Thank you," I reply.

"So the announcement came out. I've got some good and bad news. Bad news is the hospital has shut down all visitors unless you get approved for an exception. I've put your name forward because of how young you are and your situation. You need visitors. If your exception gets approved though, you only get to have two people on your list. So you have to give me the names of the people who will be your two. They won't be allowed in at the same time so they will have to work that out. I will come see you tomorrow morning to get your two names; talk to your mom about it. Let me know what you decide and hopefully by tomorrow morning we will know if it is approved for you or not," Bree says.

"My mom and I talked today. It's gonna be her and Pat; they have the flexibility to see me the most, so it's them if I get approved," I reply.

"Okay great, I'll put them down for you," Bree says.

"What about my exam tomorrow?" I panic.

"The charge nurse has approved Julia to still come in tomorrow. She will have to get screening to call up to our floor but she can still translate for you in the exam."

I sigh with relief. My professor has agreed that someone should sit with me during my exam to help with my aphasia, and to read me the questions. Between my team and me, we elected my friend Julia to come sit with me since she is also in psychology. It makes the most sense because, if I was trying to explain something, she would be the most likely to get it.

"As for the good news, Jenna ..." I look towards Bree with hope. "Day passes are still being allowed. You get to go home for Christmas Day! Go call your mom. I'll see you tomorrow."

I break out into a smile.

"Thank you Bree!" I say.

I truly do not understand Christmas at all, but the thought of going home for a day is exciting. As Bree walks out of my room, reality sets in. I am losing most of my visitors and going home for a day. What is my home? Where do I live? What exactly is this Christmas thing that everyone talks about?

Equal feelings of excitement and terror wash over me as the extent of my memory loss once again sinks in. I don't know what my home is.

I push the thoughts away and grab my phone.

"Hey Jen," my mom says as she picks up.

"Mom, I get to come home for Christmas Day."

"Are you serious Jenna? It got approved. Oh my gosh! I'm so excited, I have to tell Jordan."

My mom and I continued to debrief the day and the exciting news. I keep all the questions and nerves inside, even though I'm sure my mom can sense them. We talk until my dinner comes. I tell my mom not to worry about coming for the night. I am just going to sleep anyways, in preparation for tomorrow.

I eat my dinner while trying to calm my thoughts.

When I finish, I ask for my night meds early, get my neuro check done, and the nurses get me ready for bed.

Once they get me into bed for the night, I lay the bed flat so I can see out the top portion of the window above the construction boards covering most of the view. I start to think of all the things that exist out there. What people are doing, what it looks like, where my home is.

After a while, I grab my laptop and start researching Christmas. I learn about things such as Jesus, presents, trees, traditions, and this guy named Santa. I end up putting on a 'Christmas movie' as there are numerous lists of ones people should watch. I let my eyes close, worn out from the day, listening to stories of a man bringing children presents.

Chapter 6

December 24, 2021

The past few days have flown by in an exhausted blur, but it's settled down now.

Julia had no issues getting into the hospital to come to help me translate my exam. My rehab team and my professor had decided that I was only to write the multiple-choice section and not the short answers. At first I was bothered by this but reluctantly agreed. However, as I started writing the exam, I became happy as it was a much harder and more draining process then I thought. I am happy I accomplished it, but it was also a reminder that my brain is still quite fragile and has a lot of healing to go.

I slept for the rest of the day after finishing my exam, but the next day I hit the ground running. I told my team that I want to be in the gym as much as possible from here on out. The harder I work, the quicker I get better. I am learning there is also a balance. Pushing myself too hard actually ruins the next few days of rehab for me. I have to be careful to find that balance of pushing myself but not overdoing it.

However, as much as I am ready to hit it into high gear, the past few days are quieter than before. It is the holidays, which means staff have time off and the hospital is quiet. I have learned to dread the weekends and holidays, as they lead to boredom and sadness. Rehab is what keeps my mind occupied and tired, and without it I feel lost.

I watch social media posts of all the things happening outside the hospital world and try to soak it all in through everyone else on the weekends. My mom always tries to spend as much time as possible with me on the weekends. She also tries to arrange outside visits with others to keep me occupied, as visitors are still very restricted inside the hospital.

There is some rehab on weekends but it is normally about once, maybe twice a day if I'm lucky, and is pretty short sessions. We just do weight-bearing in my arm and leg while I play matching games or build lego patterns or such. Think of simple children's games such as in kindergarten, and that is my weekends. Activities that are simple but challenging for me.

The only other rehab on weekends is recreational therapy, which at this point consists of Christmas activities such as word searches and crosswords. I try to do them, but it doesn't end well. These activities have given me my first glimpse into the rage that I unwillingly have.

Yesterday, I was trying to complete a crossword puzzle based on the Christmas carol, Jingle Bells. However, I have zero recollection of this whole Christmas thing, let alone songs about it. Everything I know is what I have talked about with Kara in speech the past few days and what information I have collected through all the Christmas movies I watch at night.

Therefore as I was working on the crossword puzzle, I quickly became frustrated not knowing anything even though it appeared as common knowledge to everyone else. I sat and stared at the page for a while. Then all of a sudden it felt like someone took over my body. I grabbed the booklet and pencil and threw them across the room screaming "fuck you!" I pushed the table over loudly and started hitting my head off my bed rail that was beside me. And then I cried. I cried and I cried. A nurse came in after hearing the table fall. She gently picked it up without question. All she asked was, "Alone time or do you want me here?"

It was reassuring that they had experienced outbursts like this. I wrote on my speech booklet beside me 'alone.'

"Call if you need me hun," she said as she walked out.

I cried for a while and eventually fell asleep. When I woke up I was exhausted. Exhausted from emotions and scared from where that came from inside me. Emotional dysregulation was one lasting symptom of my stroke.

* * *

"Happy Christmas Eve, Jenna. Make sure you sleep tonight; you have a big day tomorrow. I'll make sure to come to you first for rounds to get you dressed and ready to go home. Have a good night, I'm headed home," my nurse says.

The nurses and I have built quite a rapport. They are all super excited for me to go home for the day. They are always excited, some of my biggest cheerleaders in here.

My mom has just gotten me ready for bed and I am all tucked in. "Okay Jen, I'm going to head home too. You need to sleep; tomorrow is going to be a crazy day for you. Ron and I are coming at 9 to get you. I will come up and grab you then. I love you so much."

"Okay Mom, I love you too. I'm excited," I reply.

After my mom leaves, I turn on a Christmas movie and get cozy into bed. I lay my bed down flat and listen to the movie as I stare at the snow falling outside the top of my window. I begin to think about what everyone is doing that night, what I know of Christmas Eve.

Mom is going home to rest and see Jordan, Pat is going to church with his family, and all the girls are at home with their families.

Later on I receive a message from Pat that says, "I just drove home from church and went by the hospital. I wanted to come in and give you a hug so badly, hun. I just keep thinking of you sitting in there all alone on Christmas Eve."

Everyone keeps saying they feel bad. But it is weird to me. I don't feel upset. I feel excited. I have no clue what this whole Christmas thing is, but I know I get to leave the hospital for a few hours tomorrow to see my family. I get to eat food besides what they serve here, I get to see all my family in the warmth instead of in the freezing cold outside, I get to learn where I live, and what my house looks like. I am getting an amazing day tomorrow. So tonight I don't feel sad, I feel uplifted.

* * *

"Good morning! Merry Christmas, happy day pass day," my nurse says as she comes in for rounds. I groggily open my eyes with a smile on my face. *I get to go home today!*

We do a neuro check which I thankfully pass so I can go home. I take my meds and wait patiently for breakfast.

"I'll come back after I finish med rounds and get you dressed kiddo," my nurse says as she leaves.

It seems like forever before breakfast comes. I eat a little bit to put something in my stomach but I remember Jordan and Logan telling me to wait for Ellen's homemade blueberry French toast bake for brunch.

After what feels like hours, my nurse comes in and gets me dressed. She turns to the chair near my bed and says, "Hey Jenna, did you see this? Santa must have come," as she holds up a wrapped gift with a label on it that says, 'To Jenna, From Santa.'

I laugh, as it is my mom's writing which I have become familiar with. "I'll open it when my Santa gets here," I say as I laugh.

Soon after I am ready, my mom strolls in. "Merry Christmas! Are you ready to see home?" she says excitedly.

"Yes! But first, what did you get me?" I ask.

My mom laughs and helps me open my gift. It is a cup, wrapped up. "Since you seem to love cups so much, we thought we would bring you one from home," my mom exclaims as she laughs. As I explained earlier, cup is an aphasia word I often use.

"Alright Jen, let's get you bundled up. Grab your dirty clothes, we can wash them today at home. Let's go! Ron is out waiting in the truck," my mom says.

We get ready and start to roll out. I sign out at the nurses' station. "Have the best day Jenna!" the charge nurse exclaims.

"Thank you! I'll see you later today," I reply, and off we go.

When we get to the main doors of the hospital, I stop rolling and look outside. "You okay?" my mom asks. I take a deep breath and tell myself I can do this. I smile at my mom and start to roll out the door to the truck.

"Hey! Nice to see you," says Ron. Between my mom, Ron, and the one good side of my body, we get me up into the truck. They fold my wheelchair into the back and Ron starts driving.

Ron and my mom try to talk to me but I have no idea what they are saying. My eyes are glued to the outside world. Soaking in everything. Trees, roads, lights, houses, buildings; everything is new.

Ron pulls into a gas station and I watch out the window, in awe of how the pump works. It is all crazy to me.

Ron gets back into the truck "Okay, before we start driving again, what music do you want on?" he asks.

"Music? I don't know," I reply.

"Well I'll pick something, but let's make it clear, repeat after me, you hate country music, you always have," Ron says.

"I hate country music," I reply.

My mom laughs loudly. And so do I, even though I am not sure why. It is just amazing to be in this truck riding along, seeing and experiencing all these new things and being filled with laughter.

The ride home passes by in a blur, and soon enough we come to a stop outside of a house. They let me sit for a moment without talking, to soak in the outside of our house.

Logan comes outside after seeing us pull up. He and Ron talk about the plan to get me inside, as it is super slippery outside and there is a step into our house. They decide to bring my chair inside first, then make footprints through the ice in the garden, and Ron will follow the footprints while carrying me inside.

We all carefully made it in safely. Once I am back in my chair, I look up and take in the house. The smells, the house itself, the people, the dogs. It is all there, all new, all amazing but extremely overwhelming.

My family makes small talk while they give me some time to soak it all in. Eventually I start to get my head around it. They give me a tour of the main floor of the house, but save the rest of the house tour for later when I've had a break. Once I am ready, they start to pull breakfast out of the oven. We eat Ellen's famous blueberry French toast bake. I can't get enough. It is real food, real coffee. It is amazing.

Everyone laughs and tells me to eat as much as I can. They all understand how bad my food had been the past month.

After breakfast, they work out how to get me downstairs. Ron carries me down while Logan brings my chair down. We turn on the wood stove and gather around on the couches. They tell me stories of my childhood and chat about their lives. I love soaking in everything they say. The morning is filled with chatting and laughing. I doze a bit on the couch, and cuddle with the dogs, as it is all a lot for me.

When I finish dozing, Ron spots me while I transfer to my wheelchair. Jordan, Logan, Ron and I begin a game of pool. Ron is on my team and he teaches me how to play. Since I only have control over my right arm, I hold the pool cue in that hand. Ron holds my left arm on the table so I can rest the cue on top of it, and I use my right hand to shoot. We play like this for quite a while until I get too tired. I like pool.

We head back to the couches to relax. "Here, try this, take a small sip," Ron says as he hands me a small glass. My mom smiles beside me.

I sip it. "I like it," I say with a smile.

"That's spiced whiskey," Ron says. He explains to me that he got a sample pack of a bunch of different whiskeys as a Christmas gift. We spend the rest of the afternoon sipping whiskey, playing pool, relaxing and chatting.

By the later afternoon I start to get tired. "We are going to have an early dinner, but would you like to have a shower here before you go back Jen, to save you for a few days there?" my mom asks.

"Yes please," I respond.

Ron and my mom find a chair to put in the shower and off we go. By now I have gotten over being vulnerable in these situations. Complete strangers have been showering and dressing me for weeks already. Having my mom shower me is nothing.

Once I'm done in the shower, my mom gets me clean pyjamas to dress in and they braid my hair. When I finish getting ready, my family all sits down to eat a wonderful ham dinner, and again I stuff myself beyond belief.

After dinner, the exhaustion of the day sets in. My family picks up on my exhaustion and they start wrapping up our visit. They all say their goodbyes as I tear up. I don't want to go back, but the day just proved how unprepared I am to leave the hospital. My mom agrees. There is no way I can function at home yet, especially without being able to walk.

My mom decides to take her car back to the hospital and my brother Andrew comes with us. The drive is a quiet one, with me fighting sleep. I still try to soak every last minute in before we get back to the hospital. When we arrive, my mom and Andrew help me into my wheelchair.

"I'll push you to the door kid; you're tired," Andrew says. He starts to push me towards the main entrance. As we approach the curb I notice Andrew isn't slowing down. He doesn't see it and I can't find the words quickly enough to warn him. Andrew pushes me straight into the curb at full force, and I go flying forward. He reaches forward and grabs me at the last moment before I fully fall out of my chair. My mom and Andrew set me back upright in my chair as we all start laughing hysterically.

"Well Jen, we almost got you back in one piece," my mom exclaims.

This began the continuous attempts of Andrew trying to ram me into curbs which he calls 'accidental.'

After our curb incident, I say goodbye to Andrew as he isn't allowed inside. My mom rolls me back up to my room and gets me into my bed. Just as she is about to leave, a loud alarm starts to go off. "Beep, Beep, Beep, Code Red, Floor 1A." Someone has set off the fire alarms.

My mom and I start laughing; it just seems to be the perfect conclusion to the day. My mom stays with me for the next half hour until the alarm stops. The nurses are unsure if we are going to have to evacuate, as it was an actual serious code. However, the fire department shows up and it eventually subsides.

"I hope you had the best day, Jenna. I loved having you home, and now we know what we need to work on to get you home permanently. Get some sleep, we will talk tomorrow, I love you," my mom says.

"I cup you Mom. Thank you," I say with a smile.

"I cup you too," my mom says as she heads out to return home with Andrew.

I quickly fall asleep, thinking about how amazing the day has been.

Chapter 7

December 29, 2021

My mom and I are hanging out in my room. She is chatting with me about her past few days. There has been some bad snow outside, so it has been a few days since I have seen her. It has been pretty quiet around here.

Bree walks into my room. "Hey! Your mom is here; I've got something I want to try. Let's head to the gym," she says. I do a pivot turn into my wheelchair, which I am getting quite good at. My mom passes me my brace and I strap it on.

The rehab team has given me an ankle foot orthosis (AFO) brace because I have drop foot on my left side when I tried to lift it. This means that the front part of my foot is difficult to lift and drags on the ground.

After putting my brace on, I grab my crocs and put them on. With the brace, plus the swelling in my foot from the nerves, my running shoes don't fit. I am getting to be known quite well in the gym because of my bright blue crocs. Everyone loves it.

When we get to the gym, Bree tells me to wheel myself up between the parallel bars. Bree and one of my physiotherapists, as well as a rehab assistant, come over and position themselves strategically around me. They help me put on a support belt. "Alright, let's start with our normal standing squats and weight bearing," Bree says. Then she looks to my mom and says "Are you ready to see Jenna take some steps?"

My mom lets out a gasp and tears up. "Yes!" she replies.

My face drops. I have been dreaming of a day when I would learn to walk again; I have been so excited. But now it is pure fear. All the things that could go wrong run through my head. "What if my leg gives out, what if I can't do it, what if I fall?" I start panicking out loud.

"Relax, you're ready, you have been getting stronger. It's time. And there are three of us here to hold you up. You will be okay," Bree says.

I try to calm down as I do my warm-up of standing and doing some squats. We do some weight shifting between my legs like we always do.

Bree then instructs me to sit and take a good break. The rehab assistant passes me water. The physiotherapist sits in front of me between the bars, while the other staff are on each of my sides. One other assistant has my wheelchair behind me for a fast sit in case something goes wrong. I feel super supported.

"Alright, whenever you are ready!" Bree says.

I take a deep breath. I start with a shaky stand. "Okay, hold there for a minute and get a feel for your legs before we start," says the physiotherapist.

I stand strong for a few seconds, then I give them a nod. "Let's do this," I say.

The rehab team grabs onto my support belt. Together Bree and I place my left hand onto the bar and I gripped the other bar with my right hand tightly. "Okay, I'm going to guide you through this," the physiotherapist says as she puts her hands on the outside of my hips. "I want you to shift your weight to the right side. Put it all into your right leg. Then slowly you are going to try and lift your left leg up and forward."

I shift my weight over into my good side. I try to lift my left leg up and my hip starts to raise. "Okay, let's bend this knee forward so you can lift without hip hiking," the physiotherapist says as she pulls my left knee forward slightly. "Good, now try again to lift that left leg."

I let my left leg go limp so my knee bends forward easily. Then I tighten it again to try and pull it up and forward. The physiotherapist guides it with her hands. Very choppily, my leg lifts up and forward to complete my first step.

"Oh Jenna," my mom exclaims as she starts tearing up.

"Okay stay focused, now comes the hard part," the physiotherapist says. "Now you need to weight shift over to your left and step forward with your right. Just remember we have you, you have the bar with your right hand for support. You're okay," she explains.

I take a shaky breath. I move my weight over to my left side. It starts shaking. The team holds my left knee and hip in place as they threaten to collapse. I lift my right foot up, my left leg starts shaking wildly, and I quickly slide my right foot forward to take a step.

The assistant brings my wheelchair up to the back of my legs. "Sit," Bree says. "That was amazing."

I look over to my mom, who is crying. "I'm so proud of you Jen," she says.

I smile back at her with tears in my eyes. Everyone just sits appreciating the moment. "Okay, how did that feel?" Bree asks after a minute.

"Terrifying but so good," I reply. "My left is definitely weak, but it felt so good. I want to be able to walk again."

"Don't worry, you will. We will get you there," Bree says.

"Okay take a minute and then let's try that once more and then we will be done for this session," says the physiotherapist.

I take a second to get my breath back to normal, surprised at how much effort that took. After a few minutes, I feel ready again. I give a firm head nod and it is all hands on deck again. I stand up feeling more sure of myself this time. The team grabs my belt, holds my left hand on the bar for me, and supports my left leg at the knee and hip. I shift my weight onto my right leg as I did before. My left knee easily bends forward and then I work to contract the muscles in my quad. My foot slowly lifts off the ground. The physiotherapist gently guides my foot forward and places it down for a step.

The team then give me more support through my belt and they hold my left knee in place to prevent collapsing. I shift my weight onto my left leg and quickly lift my right foot up and forward for another step. The process is shaky but I smile with pride. My mom is recording it while holding back tears.

I sit back down in my wheelchair and the gym erupts in applause from all the staff and other patients. "I'm proud of you, that was so good!" Bree says. "Go take a break, you deserve it. Let me know if you want to come do some arm stuff after speech today. But you've worked your leg hard enough."

"Thank you, I'm happy," I reply. The team all gives me high fives as I roll out of the gym and back to my room.

When I get back to my room my mom helps me back into my bed. "Jen I am so proud; you are doing so well," she says.

"Thank you Mom, I'm happy. I just want to walk again and get out of here," I reply.

"I know, it will come. Just keep pushing like you are and you'll be home really soon," she says.

Just then Kara from speech strolls in. "Hey Jenna, I got your new books put together. I thought we could just work through those today instead of our normal stuff," she says.

"Oh cool, okay," I reply.

Kara starts showing me my new speech books. She, my mom, and Jordan have worked on putting together a book of 'my people,' which consists of pictures of people I know from before, to relearn their faces. Kara shows it to me and we go through it together. There are pictures and then the person's name underneath. I turn to my mom and ask, "Is that you?"

My mom gives me a look of being mad and then starts laughing loudly.

"That's you but not you. That is like a clone, like the sheep. There's a clone sheep of you, Mom," I say with confusion.

Through laughter my mom says, "No, that is your Uncle Mark; that is not me."

It turns out that everyone calls my mom and Uncle Mark twins because they look almost identical, but they are not in fact twins. They always think it is hilarious when people call them twins or get them mixed up. So anytime anyone hears this story about me calling Mark my mom, they think it is hilarious.

After going through some of my people, Kara shows me another book they made for me, which is an 'all about me' book. Jordan and my mom have given Kara a bunch of information about me so I can relearn who I was. We talk about me growing up being a competitive dancer and a baseball player, we discuss where I was born, and all the places I have lived so far. Big life events that have happened, family vacations I've gone on. We even go over things I have no idea about, like my favourite restaurant, my favourite food, and the foods I don't like. All the things about me, big and small.

This is really interesting for me to learn. I feel closer to myself but also more of a stranger at the same time. It is like learning about someone I have never met before, except I am inside their body. I have been to a place called Costa Rica? I was born in Guelph? I loved something called camping, I could dance, I liked reading, the water was a deep connection to me? All these things, all my thoughts swirl in my head.

It is like I am listening to a song playing loudly around me. I can feel the rhythm in my body, the rhythm of me, but the lyrics, the memories, the feelings are being drowned out. I can almost taste who I was, but it is so far out of my grasp at the same time. 21 years of my life floating out there for everyone else to experience, remember, reflect on. But I know none of it except for the past three weeks.

These feelings haven't hit me like they are now. I haven't fully grasped how much I am missing, how much everyone else knows. I have been learning the alphabet, words, common objects, the seasons, the months of the year. I knew I was missing this information. But wow, is there more to it! I don't even know me. Where do I begin to find me again? How do you re-learn 21 years of your life, 21 years of memories, 21 years of knowing other people?

21 years, gone in one day.

I am a foreigner in my own world. A foreigner in my own brain, in my own body, in my own life. And now I have to begin to find myself.

"Let's stop there for today," Kara says as she and my mom can see the emotions hitting me. She leaves my room and my mom gives me a minute to digest everything.

My head starts to hurt, and the panic starts to settle in. What was my life like before? Who was I? The questions start swirling out of control.

"Close your eyes, rest. We have tons of time to relearn this stuff," my mom says.

I put in my headphones to listen to my new favourite thing I have learned, called Spotify. I do what my mom said, I close my eyes and work to calm down. My mom gives me a hug and heads out. "I'll be back later. Take some you time."

My mom is quite good at knowing when I need to be alone because the world is too much. I listen to music and push the panic away for a while.

* * *

I hear my door creak open so I open my eyes. Pat is here. “Hey hun, how are you feeling?” he asks.

“I’m okay, tired now,” I respond, as I am sure he and my mom talked about my overwhelming time an hour ago. He comes by my bed and starts asking me about how everything is going. I take some time to show him my new speech books. Then I remember earlier. I stop and look at him, and a smile breaks out on my face. “Babe, guess what?” I say.

“What?” he asks with a smile.

“Wait, did my mom tell you already?” I say, feeling disappointed.

“No, she said I had to ask you what you did earlier but she wouldn’t tell me anything, just said it was exciting,” he says.

“I took steps, I walked,” I say loudly with a huge smile.

“What!?! No way,” he replies as he grabs me into a hug. “I’m so sorry I missed that. Oh wow, that’s amazing, I’m so proud of you!” he says with the biggest smile on his face.

"Thank you. My mom will send you the video. I'm sure you will see me in action later too," I say.

Pat and I continue talking for a while, both of us excited about my recovery so far. The panic feelings from before are pushed to the back of my mind for later.

Not long after Pat gets there, Bree comes into my room. "Hey, you wanna go to the gym once more before the end of the day?" she asks.

"Yeah!" I reply.

Pat spots me while I pivot into my wheelchair and off we all go to the gym. Once we get there Bree tells me to wheel to the back so we can do some arm work. She goes into the closet and comes out with a weird board with wheels. She sets it on the table in front of me. "Okay, we call this a skateboard. So we are going to strap your left arm into it and try to get you to move your arm, kinda like windshield wipers," she says as she shows me the motion.

I pick up my left arm with my right hand and place it into the skateboard thing. Bree straps my arm in. I take a deep breath and try to move my arm. My fingers start to move a little, followed slowly by my wrist from side to side. It becomes quite shaky.

"Okay, take a breath," Bree says.

I take a minute before trying again. Again my fingers and wrist have some small movements but my arm is not moving as a whole.

Bree puts her hand on my shoulder as it starts to lift upwards. "Try to move the arm and not the shoulder. Good, keep trying," she says.

"Wait, stop," she exclaims and I stop. She wraps her hand around my bicep. "Okay, try again." I take a breath, focus myself, and try to get some movement.

"Ahh, Jenna! I think I know the problem," Bree claims with excitement. "The problem isn't your arm not working at all, it's working too much! Your bicep, which is this front muscle, and your tricep here in the back are both being turned on at the same time, working against each other," Bree explains. "We just need to figure out how to turn one on and one off so they aren't working against each other."

This is such a big discovery, as up till now, we could not understand why I was getting hardly any movement in my arm. It gives me hope that we can start to get my arm working again.

Bree starts running through possible solutions "Starting tomorrow let's try some electromagnetic stimulation on your arm as you do your exercises, as well as some band work. I'll ask the rest of the rehab team if they have any ideas at all. If we can't get it to work, there are options like botox to settle some of the muscles. But don't worry yet, let's try some different methods first."

"Okay" I say, starting to get excited about getting somewhere.

"That was a lot to take in for today. Why don't we stop there and next time Pat comes back we can show him your new skills you learned earlier?" Bree says with a wink.

"I heard about them! I cannot wait to see them!" Pat says, and I smile.

"Before we finish though, can I ask you something?" Pat says to Bree.

"Yeah of course," she replies.

"Jenna and her mom and I have been talking a bit about what the long-term plan is. She has been in here for around a month so far. How long do you see her here? Like what is this looking like?" Pat asks.

"Yeah, good questions. So looking at where you are at right now Jenna, I would say the earliest you will be out of here is end of January, which is next month. The problem is there is very limited rehab outside the hospital due to Covid, your age, and not having a solid diagnosis. So if you get discharged then you get no therapy and that would be detrimental to your recovery at this point. As well, we talked about how hard Christmas Day was at home. It was a lot and your house isn't set up for you to be there. Plus there is a shortage of home care nurses so that would put all your showers, dressing, food, bathroom stuff on your family, which is a lot," Bree says as I nod. "So I'm thinking late January, February at the earliest, unless we can get you a spot in outpatient rehab. But it is also the holidays still. Let's set that as a tentative timeline and after the holidays and rehab is back to normal schedule we can do an assessment and set a discharge plan and date to work towards," Bree explains.

"Okay." I nod, feeling a bit upset with such a long time still expected in the hospital.

"That sounds like what I had in mind; you okay?" Pat asks me.

"Yeah, just taking it in," I say.

"Okay great work today. Let me know if you need anything else," Bree says.

"Thanks," I say as Pat and I roll back to my room.

"You'll get home hun. Think about it, you took steps this morning, you'll be walking by next week. You've got this," Pat says.

"I know, just frustrating," I say, not wanting to discuss it anymore.

"Hey, I brought you something for Christmas," he says, to get my attention off the news.

Pat passes me a bag. I pull out a massage gun. "Because you are always so sore from not being able to get up," Pat says.

I smile. "Flip over onto your stomach in your bed, hun," he says.

I have started doing a new thing that he likes to call 'tummy time.' My back and butt are always hurting from sitting/lying down constantly. So I take time to lie on my stomach and extend my right side to try and stretch out a bit on my bed. I roll onto my stomach and he shows me how the massager works on my back. It feels nice and less stiff. This quite quickly will become a daily routine of massaging out my back and butt to be less stiff, especially with my arthritis.

Once I am done stretching, Pat helps me flip back over on my bed to sit up. We start talking about random stuff, his work, his day, anything and everything. We always have the best conversations. I start to get tired, so my speech starts to dwindle. As well, my filter skills really go away when I get tired. I will say random things that make no sense or just random things that pop into my head that have no relevance to the conversation. My family/friends and I have coined this behaviour as 'stroke brain.'

For example, the last time I saw Pat, we somehow got onto this conversation where he told me about this lady who was accused of murdering her child because it went missing while camping. It turns out that a wild dingo stole her baby and ate it. I had watched video reports on it and thought it was so strange but also funny because I didn't understand what it really meant. But things like this stuck with me. So often when I would get 'stroke brain' I would randomly call people 'fucking dingos.' I would just yell out, 'A dingo ate my baby. You're a fucking dingo.' It is kind of hilarious.

So as Pat was in the middle of telling me about his Christmas Day, I just yell, 'Ah you're a fucking dingo,' and we both burst into laughter.

Once I start to have stroke brain, Pat can tell I am tired. He tells me I should take some rest time and go to bed. I agree without arguing for once. We say our goodbyes and I settle in for the night after a very good, but very emotional day.

Chapter 8

January 3, 2022

"I'm sorry, no visitors, no leaving your room, no gym time. It's for your safety," the hospitalist says. I watch him leave my room; he puts a hazardous waste bin inside my doorway. A nurse comes over and tapes up two huge 'Stop. Hazardous. Infected" signs outside my room. She gives me a sad look and swings my door closed. Darkness and tears wash over me. I am isolated. Inside this room, the only four walls I will see for the next 10 days. I put my bed down so I can lie flat. I stare out the top slit of my window watching the snow fall outside as the tears fall down my face.

It is day three of isolation. The boredom has set in hard. I am confined to my room. No visitors. Limited rehab as they aren't allowed to bring things into my room or take me out to the gym. I am spending my days watching Netflix, staring out the little window slit I have, and watching the rat that lives between my window and the wood boarding it up. I have tried to do some of my own exercises but am quickly losing motivation as I still need to be spotted to do anything. I try to facetime friends whenever possible but even the motivation is falling away for that. I eat cold food and have to strategically plan my bathroom times. The nurses have to fully gown up before coming in so it takes a while for them to come help me. The food staff aren't allowed in my room. They place my tray of food on the floor outside my door and I wait for a nurse to gown up and bring it to me. I am told this is for my safety. My tests are still negative. But I am being kept safe, they say. I am turning numb. Isolated, alone, numb.

Today is day four of isolation. My rehab team recognizes I'm not okay. They come in for a bit each day to get me moving now. It's awkward. They are fully gowned, n-95 mask with another medical mask on top, goggles and a shield on. I can't hear them, they can't hear me. I can't see their face, they can't safely see me out of their fogged goggles and shield. They brought me a walker and I've been able to slowly walk with them helping me, and the walker. But it doesn't bring me joy. How do I feel joy when I'm alone, when my mom or Pat can't even share these moments with me?

Today Bree came in and changed my rehab sheet. She updated my bathroom, dressing and eating requirements from all red (full assistance) to yellow (some assistance) because the nurses are so crazy with a whole floor in isolation that it takes them up to an hour to come help me. I told Bree I didn't care if I fell; I was figuring out how to do more on my own. She said that was fair enough.

So as much as this isolation is sucking the joy out of me, it's forcing me to figure out how to be more independent.

Kara came to do speech today. Normally she sits outside my room and we yell across the room at each other so I can actually hear her without three masks and a face shield in the way. I watch other people say words and listen to their pronunciation to learn how to say them myself. So three masks interrupting that makes it hard. But today she walked up to me as I was crying. Kara told me to hold on. She was gone for a few minutes but then returned fully gowned up. She entered my room and helped me to my wheelchair. She said speech was canceled for the day and she was just there to be my friend. We talked for a bit. I cried. She asked if I wanted my hair braided. It was gross and bothering me. I had gone over a week without a shower since I wasn't allowed to use the shower rooms across the hall and my room had no hot water. If only I had known I would be isolated, I would've made sure to shower the day before. But seeing Kara was nice, she just talked about other things to distract me, and braided my hair. When she had to leave she promised me she would be back tomorrow to do the same. She said she would be my friend in here.

Besides this small moment, what is joy anymore?

Today is day six.

I wake up to my first period since my stroke. I have bled through my pants overnight. My sheets are bloody. I wake up and cry. I feel disgusting. I was already gross and now I have blood all over me and no way to clean it up.

My nurse comes in to get me out of bed. She walks into the room and I burst into tears. I tell her I don't want to be here anymore. That I can't do this. That I want a shower. I want my mom. I want Pat. I want my family. I want to get back to therapy. I want to be okay again.

She holds me and lets me cry. I cry for a while.

Then without talking she slowly starts to help me out of bed. When I get up, we both look at the puddle of blood that is under me and I start sobbing harder.

My nurse looks me in the eye and says, "Fuck this, get your stuff, we are going for a shower."

She walks into my bathroom and tries to run the water; of course it won't get warm even though the hospital claims it will. My nurse turns to me and says, "I wouldn't shower my dog in this water, let alone you. I don't care. This is bullshit." She grabs my shower chair and helps me onto it. We roll over to the doorway. She opens the door and steps out to look around. "Clear," she says with a smile and pushes me across the hallway into the shower room. When we get in there she starts the hot water.

It is the best shower of my life. I cry happy tears in the shower. When we are done, she sneaks me back into my room and changes my sheets. I feel a small piece of joy again.

Today is day seven of isolation. I'm still testing negative. The higher ups of the hospital still say this is for my safety. My nurse again tells me this is bullshit. She let my mom come sit outside my door today. My nurse had found me crying for the seventh day on the phone to my mom, saying I want to go home. That I hate life. That I can't do this. I'm missing so much rehab time that I need. My nurse told my mom to come sit at my door while gowned up. It is amazing to have her here. But when my mom goes to leave, I lose it. The uncontrollable sobs start. I'm crying and screaming that I can't do this anymore. My mom starts to cry, and tries to calm me down. I scream as my neighbour screams for help. His screams drive me nuts; he is delusional and screams all day for the nurses. The sympathy has left my body. It adds to my sobs. The charge nurse comes by as she hears my sobs and the patient's screams next to me. She witnesses my mom and me crying. She stops and looks around. She gives my mom a once over in her gown, and hands her a face shield and pair of gloves. Confused, my mom puts them on. The nurse looks at us both and says, "Go give your daughter a hug or I will. I can't do this to her anymore."

"Are you serious?" my mom asks.

The nurse gently guides my mom inside my room and closes the door quickly. As she shuts the door, she says, "Don't open this door; do not tell anyone we did this."

My mom is able to hug me. I am negative, I don't have the virus, she is wearing so much PPE I'm not even sure it is my mom. The nurses can be fired for this, but this is for my 'safety,' they say.

Today is day nine of isolation. My mom's hug didn't last as long as I hoped it would. Tomorrow was supposed to be day ten of isolation and then freedom. Bree just informed me that my isolation has been extended at least another three days for no known reason. I am still negative, the nurse that had Covid is my nurse again tomorrow, back from her isolation period, yet mine is extended again.

The tears are back. The sobs to my mom. I was so close to being outside again. So close to being okay. Yet it's all being sucked away again.

Yesterday someone died from a stroke on my floor. Their family wasn't allowed in to see them, even though the doctors knew they weren't going to make it. The patient didn't have Covid but they were isolated just like me. They died alone. Their family had no choice but to be arrested for fighting security to get inside the hospital or let them die alone. What kind of world are we living in?

My mom told me to type out my feelings today. I'm struggling with my words again. I feel gross without a shower again. I'm in a hard struggle with this life.

She told me to write it out and send it to her.

When she read it, she told me it was beautiful. That it should be shared. That people need to know about these conditions. That I should fight. I ask her how. She explains social media and the possible power in it. She tells me it might make me feel better and less alone.

Jordan calls and walks me through how to post something like my words onto social media. I post my story. And now I stare at the small slit of a window and dream of getting out of here until I fall asleep.

* * *

Today is day ten. I was supposed to be out of isolation today. I am not.

My phone is going off like crazy. I grab it off my table and unlock it. Wait. What is happening? I look at my notifications. Over 1000 of them. I quickly call Jordan. "What is happening?" I ask. They look on my instagram and facebook. My posts have blown up overnight. I'm confused, unsure, scared what this means. Jordan explains the anger, the fear for me, the empathy, the shared experiences, the rage in others about my story. They explain that my story is out there, that it has become a bigger thing than I know. That people support me, that I am not alone. That they needed to hear this. That I have a fire burning within me.

My posts continue to get acknowledgment by people. People across Canada, across the world. News stations contact me, strangers reach out to me, to my family, my friends. I have random people send me books to read, slippers to be comfy, snacks to keep me happy. The president of Trent University sends me a care package. But not a single politician joins the conversation. Thousands of tags on my posts, but locally, provincially, and federally I am ignored.

It speaks volumes to me. It speaks volumes to my new cheerleaders.

This is my first insight into the shambles of our current world. The shambles of this situation. But for once over the past week or so, I don't feel quite so alone.

My care team rallies alongside me. They secretly thank me for my post and say they want to support it but will lose their job if they do. I've been told the hospital is not impressed with me. They claim I am exacerbating my issues. They say I am allowed showers as there is running water, yet those who actually work on my floor have deemed it too cold. I am given food on the normal schedule, the hospital proclaims, yet they don't care to see or help the nurses who have to individually gown up and help feed all ten of their patients which turns a normal hour long job into six hours. They don't come to see my rehab go from hard work every possible second, to twenty minutes a day. They aren't here, yet they have a lot to say about me.

These next few days scream volumes to me about our world. The hospital executives come out with some new guidelines for my care team. They give them approval to gown me and themselves up, and wheel me outside for ten minutes each morning and afternoon so I can see outside. They allow my team to bring me to sit at a window if we all wear strict PPE for ten minutes a day, so I can't keep saying I have no sunlight exposure. They do all kinds of things to get me to shut up.

People are messaging me, saying they will pay for therapy outside the hospital for me. A local business offered to start a go-fund-me and to help make my house wheelchair accessible so I can go home. But I deny it all. I keep saying, so I leave and then what? The man next to me who died alone didn't get these opportunities. I leave and I get my family. Everyone else in here won't. This isn't about me. This is about this whole situation. I lost my voice during my stroke but I've found it again and I will not stop using it.

* * *

The hospital soon realizes that I am not going to back down from the news and the energy. They are pretty quick to get me out of isolation. After 13 days I am freed from my room, but the rest of the floor around me is not. Because they do not have a voice, I am their voice, but I am not able to do it for them. The world has moved on to the next problem; my time has passed.

It saddens me that I went through this. The hospital has changed its policies in regard to allowing for some visitors if people are testing negative. However, they weren't easy to change. I had no effect on the world policies, as politicians found it easy to ignore me. I am surprised at this. At the lack of care. Trent University was able to send me a care package, yet the local Peterborough MPP was not able to answer my countless emails, tags and direct messages along with thousands of other people's. But I try not to focus on the negatives. I try to focus on the people who did care, those who still reach out to me asking how I am. Those who share my story, check in on me, and fight my fight with me.

Over thirteen days of being negative for Covid, thirteen days of isolation, thirteen of the worst days of my life that I've known, but I learned how everyday people can come together in support. I learned how deeply my hospital team cares for me. I learned how loved I am. I learned that my speech maybe isn't great, that my left side is still a struggle to move, that I know so little about the world, but over top of all that, I have a powerful voice. One that I must use to share my story. And that is what I continue to do.

Chapter 9

January 15, 2022

I wake up to my night nurse calling my name. She passes me a piece of paper, which says "Hip hip hooray, you come out of isolation today," and she has coloured in the balloons around it. "I wanted to give this to you before shift change," she says as she congratulates me. I feel butterflies in my stomach. Today I get a shower. Today I get to hit the gym hard and get back onto my end of January discharge plan. Today is a good day.

And it is. My team brings me outside early in the morning to experience the air. I get to feel winter hit my skin without a mask, gown or gloves on. I get to breathe it in.

The gym cheers and celebrates when I roll back in. Everyone is so happy to see me outside of my room. Bree and I have a couple of good sessions, with me walking between the bars and with a walker. We notice some lack of stamina from before, but she says it will come back quickly; we just have to build it back up. She tells me that once my stamina is back we are going to try walking with a cane, and then walking with nothing. Walking independently and walking up and down stairs are our next goals.

We are still using electrostimulation on my arm. I am starting to get more control over my arm. We are still having issues with my muscles all turning on at once but I am learning how to make my arm work regardless. My fingers are starting to be able to grip things, which is nice as I can actually hold things in my hand for a few seconds before they fall.

My speech is also improving. I am able to hold conversations and say the words I want to say. I still experience aphasia, dysfluency, and a lack of knowledge of words, but I am much better than I was in the early days of December.

My memory is still a struggle. I think of my brain like a towel, soaking up all the water of information people give to me. I am hungry for knowledge, as it appears I lack so much.

I have begun deep diving into my psychology work as my classes have started up again. I have a thesis to relearn and then finish. I have two other classes as well. And I also can't wait to get back to being a research assistant in the cognition lab at school.

The semester is working out well for me because, as a result of Covid, classes are online for the time being. Therefore I don't have to put my last semester on hold while I am still hospitalized (even though my nurses and team think I am crazy). It is nice to have learning built into my routine.

I am feeling positive about where I am. I enjoy the busyness of my routine, especially now that I am allowed to do outside visits again with my family and friends. We are also beginning to talk about going home. Bree had to set a discharge date as per policy, and we agreed on January 28, 2022.

The date is hung on my patient whiteboard with all my other information. Every morning when I wake up, I look to it and read the date. Then I open my calendar and count how many more days I have to prepare.

The days are passing quickly, and I have mixed emotions. I am so excited to go home. But the hospital is all I know. I have been home for one day. Eight hours outside of this building is all I can remember about the outside world.

On one of my recent dives through the internet, I learned about correctional facilities. I find them fascinating. One part in particular has stuck with me: sometimes when people get released from prison, they purposefully commit crimes so they can be placed back in jail. Life outside of jail is too much for them; they don't know how to live in a world they feel they don't belong in, and don't understand.

I connect with these ideas. I have a vision of me getting discharged from the hospital, my home, what I know. I will return to my old life, that I know nothing about. I will go back to school and re-meet my friends, and professors and supervisors that I don't even know anymore. I will go back to my house with my mom and learn how to cook and do laundry again. I will eventually move back to the house I rent in Peterborough, and will have to relearn how to be independent. I will go to the stores my friends talk about, such as Costco. But I am worried my head will explode. What if it is all too much? What if I can't do it? There is no way to re-check myself into the hospital. No way to make myself have another stroke to forget the scariness of the outside world. I have to face it whether I want to or not, and that is a petrifying thought.

I broke down the other night when Bree told me my tentative discharge date. She saw the panic in my eyes when she told me, but quickly reassured me that we could always postpone it if I wasn't ready when the time came. I then cried to my mom, who reminded me that it was going to be okay. "But Mom, what if my head just like explodes with trying to fit everything in?" I asked. "What if someone talks to me and I stutter? What if someone isn't in my 'people book' and I don't know who they are and they hate me? What if people think I'm stupid because I don't know what something is? What if I can't do it? This place, these people, this is my home, these are my friends. How do I just leave my best friend Bree, or her student, or Kara and Sarah, or the nurses? How do I just leave? What if I'm not ready?" I cried out.

"Jen, take a breath. You are going to leave here; they want to see you grow. It will be time and you will be okay. We are here to help you. You will panic. You will have awkward moments. People won't think you are stupid; people will get it. Remember how supportive people are of your posts. You will be okay. Your friends will understand, and your professors will understand. Just explain what happened and ask them to introduce themselves again. We are all here together to make this okay for you. Because you are one of the strongest, most brilliant, fucking dingos that I know, and you will be fine outside these walls," my mom replied.

It was encouraging.

Deep down I know I will be fine, but getting to the part where I am fine might be hard.

The panic has caused me to hit things into high gear. Over the next few days, I work harder than I had before. I breathe in every second of the gym I can. I read and work to memorize my 'about me' and 'people' books multiple times a day. I Google my supervisors and professors from Trent University to memorize their faces so I don't look dumb. I practice holding conversations as best as I can. And I begin to walk unassisted.

* * *

Bree gets me to roll up between the bars as I always do for our warm-ups. However, this time she turns to my mom and says "You're going to want to record this." Then she looks to me and says "Let's walk."

I smile at my mom, who smiles back. I give my team a reassuring smile to make me feel more confident.

"Okay just like you have been doing but this time don't hold the bars. You are so ready for this!" Bree says. We have been practicing putting less pressure on the bars lately.

I stand up from my wheelchair and nod to signify that I am ready. I let go of the bar with my right hand, my left just dangles at my side.

I focus on the motions. I put all my weight into my right leg. I let my left knee go limp so it bends forward at a 90-degree angle. I squeeze my left quad as hard as I can to get it to engage and I lift it upwards. I shakily move my foot forward and downwards to complete a step. The placement of my foot isn't great, but the physiotherapist shifts it back to a straight position. I fall a little to the side as my balance is off, but the team holds my support belt strongly.

I begin to focus on holding my left leg strong as I put my weight into it. I lift my right leg and quickly take a step.

The gym is silent. I focus back on my left leg with my weight shifted into my right leg and repeat the stepping motions. Limp, bend, engage, lift, forward, down, sturdy. I complete another step with my left foot. I take another step with my right and then motion to sit.

I feel the wheelchair pushed gently up against the back of my legs signaling it's ready for me. I sit in my wheelchair and look up as a roar of applause and cheers breaks out in the room.

I look to my mom; her face is streaked with tears and her huge smile matches mine.

I just walked! I walked on my own! I took four steps on my own! I just fucking walked!

The room quiets down slowly. Bree smiles at me. "I did it!" I say.

Again the room breaks out into cheers and laughter. "Yeah you did!" Bree says.

I feel adrenaline rush through my body. I feel like I can do anything. I turn to my rehab team and say "Let's do it again."

And we do. Again and again and again. I continue to take a few steps, rest, a few steps, rest, until my legs can no longer lift me anymore.

I ask if we can practice walking every day. My rehab team laughs and promises me we can keep doing it anytime I want.

I have found the drug of walking and I am addicted.

* * *

It's been a week since I took those first unassisted steps. I have come so far already. I am now walking with a cane. I do laps of walking around the nurses station with Bree walking beside me and her student pushing my wheelchair behind me for those well-needed breaks.

I hate using the cane. It makes me feel undignified, old, and embarrassed. But it allows me to walk so I suck it up and use it. It gives me support outside of the parallel bars in case I need to lean into something.

Bree says I am almost ready to ditch it, she just wants me to build a little more strength. I keep on pushing.

"So I'm thinking this afternoon we try the stairs," Bree says as we finish our morning laps.

"Yes please," I reply with great excitement. Being able to walk up and down stairs puts me one step closer to getting home (pun intended).

Home is right around the corner and, as scared as I am, I am also excited. I have begun to recognize that a life inside this hospital will become even more boring as time goes on. And the longer I hold a bed on this floor, the more time I am taking from someone else who needs these people's help. I have found my motivation to get out of here; I miss my people, and I miss exploring more of life.

I am also getting more excited about leaving because it is becoming more real. This Saturday coming up, I have a day pass approved to go home for the day. It is kind of like a trial run to see what is still a struggle and what the house needs in order to work for me. Ron has bought a bunch of assistive stuff like grab bars to place in our house for me. He wants me there to install them, however, because anyone who knows us is aware that Ron and I don't exactly share the same height. Where he would need to grab to get off the toilet wouldn't be ideal for me.

So I get to go home and ensure the house is ready. It will also be an opportunity for me to see if there are any last-minute skills Bree and I need to work on to make my home life easier.

My family is excited to get me home for the day and then to get me home permanently. It has been a long couple of months of outside visits and just overall stress. It is time I go home.

Chapter 10

January 28, 2022

My mom has just put the last bag of stuff into the car. All that is left is for me to leave. I look around one last time. I check the closet to make sure it is empty. I say goodbye to the rat in the window. I reflect on my gratitude that I never have to deal with the crappy shower again. I smile, thinking how far I have come since my first days here. I remember the anger I've experienced in here. I remember the laughter I've shared. The good times and the bad. I scan the room one last time, take a big deep breath and nod to my mom. "Let's go," I say.

I shut the door to the room that was mine for the past two months, nervous but ready to leave.

I start to walk down the hall towards the nurses' station, towards the outside world. My mom follows me close behind, with my wheelchair ready in case I need it.

I walk by the empty desk. *That's strange,* I think. I turn the corner towards the ward doors.

The hallway explodes with clapping, cheering and shouts. Everyone is here; the nurses, the physiotherapists, the occupational therapists, my speech team, the wife of patient J, and Bree. I start crying as I walk. The clapping gets louder.

Bree steps out of line and grabs me into a huge hug. "You've got this, you are so ready!" she says. She steps back and I pull her in again with my right arm. "Thank you so much," I choke out. Her eyes light up with a smile under her mask and she gives me a look of sureness, sure that I can do this, sure that I will be okay. I walk strongly to the end of the hallway, the end of the line of my support team, and turn around.

With tears streaming down my face I take one last look at the faces, the people who got me here, my closest friends for the last 49 days. I wave and yell thank you over their cheers and applause.

Then I turn and continue the rest of my walk out to my mom's car.

On the car ride home, my mom and I sit in silence. She driving, me processing through the exhaustion of the morning and the preparation to get here. I almost fall asleep in the car but force myself to stay awake and soak in everything that blurs by the window.

My mom pulls the car into the driveway. She turns and looks at me. She looks like she wants to say something but we both know there are no words to describe this moment. There is no limit on my time home today before I have to go back. It's not a day pass, this is a forever now. 49 days in the hospital, 49 days of the hardest work of my life, 49 days of emotions, 49 days of outside visits, and now I'm home. We smile at each other and she gets out of the car. Jordan comes outside and holds my left side as I shuffle to the door. We get inside and I collapse on the couch in pure exhaustion.

Jordan and Mom carry in all my stuff from the car. Once my wheelchair is inside I transfer into it and wheel over to the bed. We've decided that I will sleep in my mom's bed for now. Her room is on the main floor with the kitchen and bathroom. This way I don't have to worry about the stairs until I'm stronger.

I transfer to the bed and very quickly fall asleep.

My dreams have served me as a place for reflection and learning. I dream about things that I have no memories of, and when I wake I quickly try to Google everything in those dreams. They have led me to so much learning.

For example, I had a dream about being locked in a gas chamber when I was in the hospital. I woke up very confused about what a gas chamber was. I didn't even know that it was called a gas chamber at the time. But a deep internet search led me to learn about many things, including gas chambers, the tragedy of the Holocaust, what war is, a man named Hitler, and religion. I began to ask questions about these events, and my friends and family explained them. It is mind-blowing. I was so confused when they told me that Hitler has been dead for years. I don't understand the concept of the past or death. How did things happen before me? How are people older than me? There are people that have died? Time is a concept I struggle with.

On this particular day after returning home from the hospital, I dream of reflection. I dream of the past two weeks and how hard I have worked, how worthwhile it all will be. I dream of the exhaustion, the draining feelings, and the excitement.

In the past two weeks, I have done a lot, and pushed harder in rehab than I had over the past two months. I have mastered how to do stairs. I can do them without hands-on assistance, rather just a spotter. I hold the rail with my right hand and take them one step at a time.

I can walk for short distances without any support. I have learned to walk on the pavement outside and not just on the hospital floor. I have even started to experience walking on grass in the past few days. I have started learning how to walk in winter boots instead of my crocs or running shoes. But this is a work in progress.

Last week I started walking with ski poles. It was a challenge at first to even be able to hold the pole in my left hand, but once I had enough strength to keep it in my hand, Bree grabbed the other end and we used them to make my arms swing while I walked. Otherwise, my left arm just sits dead at my side while I walk. I am slowly getting some natural swing back in my arm.

I also got to do an assessment with Blake, my outpatient physiotherapist, who will be booking me in to do an official assessment within the next few weeks. He is a kind and funny guy who I am looking forward to working with.

All of the hard work feels worth it. Because here I am dreaming in my own home, outside the hospital.

* * *

It is Monday and, since coming home on Friday, I have mostly just rested and gotten used to my new surroundings. I've had a few simple cooking lessons, such as how to boil water, how to cut vegetables (which was a learning curve with only one good hand) and even how I can just choose whatever food I want from the pantry and fridge. Being home is mind-blowing, and I love learning it all. It's a whole world that I had no idea existed.

Earlier today I met with my new home care occupational therapist. She came out to the house and did an assessment. I found her very nice, but not the most helpful. She listened but didn't seem to get my situation. I found it to be lots of advocating for myself.

When she assessed the house, she was impressed with the accessibility changes we had already made. She also had a few additional supports she wanted to add.

She told me that I could use a sling for my left arm when needed, to take off the weight of it hanging from my shoulder. It could also hold my arm in a position that makes my hand accessible to use when there is nothing to lean it on. For example, when cutting a cucumber, I can have my arm in a sling and use my left hand to try and hold the cucumber so I can cut with my right hand. I appreciated the suggestion.

She then encouraged me to get bed rails so I could get myself out of bed more easily, but I declined. I don't find it much of a challenge and I already feel dumb with the changes to my house.

When we got to my mobility aids, I found it frustrating. Her recommendation was to use a walker instead of a wheelchair so I could practice walking more. However, the wheelchair is more beneficial to me with good reason. I use the wheelchair when I am tired from walking but also when my surroundings are too much in my head. When I get tired, when it is too busy, when it is hard to solely focus on walking, or when there is going to be a lot of people and I may get bumped, I use my wheelchair. The OT said I could use a walker for all of that. If I got tired, I could just sit down for a while and then continue. I explained how this could become impractical. What if I need to get to class in ten minutes; how am I supposed to just sit for an hour before going? I had to argue my case for a while before I just said I was firm in my decision to keep the wheelchair. She eventually saw I was not going to change my mind, and gave up for this visit.

After our home assessment, she did offer me some supports for my cognitive deficits. She recommended many apps that I could download to work on my memory, dual-tasking, and overall mental stimulation. I found this helpful. When the assessment was done, I was exhausted, so I napped. It is funny how such seemingly little things take the biggest toll on me.

These assessments are quickly becoming my new normal. On Friday this week I am scheduled to go to my outpatient stroke physiotherapy assessment. I am so grateful to have this opportunity. Bree had advocated strongly for me to have a spot on the waitlist. Since my stroke isn't confirmed and I am so young, I don't really meet the criteria for the program. However, nowhere else in this area will take me except normal physiotherapy. Those could be beneficial; however, the hospital program is specialized in neurological physio, which makes a huge difference for my recovery. As well, all the programs outside the hospital are private and, as a student who hasn't worked since November, I have no money to spare. Therefore it is like winning the lottery that I got into the outpatient stroke program and that a spot has opened so fast.

I have also recently gotten an assessment for the Xolair program for my mast cell disorder. My doctors and I had been working for months prior to my stroke to try and get my mast cell under control. We have finally received government approval to start the Xolair program, which is a medicinal injection. I received my first Xolair shot a couple weeks ago and so far so good. I did react slightly to the shot by being seemingly high and then super exhausted and lethargic the next day. However, my throat did not close. I haven't had an anaphylactic reaction since before my stroke, so this is all looking positive.

With all the assessments comes excitement, but also a craving to get back to a 'normal' life. A life I can't even remember, but I crave.

"Jen, you have to give yourself some time. We will get you back there as soon as possible, but you need to take some time. You haven't even been home for more than three days. You haven't even gone out, you haven't gone to class. Take a breath," my mom says.

"I know, but I'm missing out on so much. I want to be back at my Peterborough house. I want to be with the girls. I want to be normal again," I cry.

"And you will be. You will be back before you know it, but you have to chill a bit. Let's see how this week goes, how class goes tomorrow. Then we can make a game plan," she says.

I want to move back to my own house so badly, and it has only been a weekend since my release from the hospital.

I miss my friends, I miss my independence, I just want to feel normal.

I am terrified to go to class tomorrow. To show my face to all those that know me, but I have no recollection of them. To show up to an inaccessible campus that I've been warned about. To show up in front of my peers in a wheelchair. It is daunting to not remember anyone, to not remember your school and to know that everyone will stare.

My friend from class is going to meet me and my mom outside the building. Bella also said she will meet me. My mom will drop me off, and Bella and my friend are going to take me into the school. They will show me where the elevator is, and get me settled in my classroom. My friend has promised to sit with me in class, and Bella is going to study while waiting for me outside the classroom. Bella is then going to drive me home.

Knowing that Bella is going to show up makes me feel like I might get through it. I literally cannot think of having to go tomorrow without wanting to throw up. But Bella gives me some reassurance as she will be there any time I need her. She is the greatest support I can imagine for this. Which is partly why I want to get back to living with her and the other girls. They treat me like normal, like one of them, but also know my limits and when to make me rest. They make me feel like just Jenna. Not Jenna who had a stroke and is now disabled.

Chapter 11

February 2022

The first month home is a whirlwind. I survive my first in-person class of the term. I am so grateful for my friends, as it is probably the hardest thing I have done so far, fear-wise. But I get through it. I have major feelings of anxiety going to school but I push through and continue because I want my degree so badly.

My life has taken a focus on re-experiencing and re-learning the world. Everyone wants to re-meet me, to do things with me and show me the world.

Jordan and Andrew took me skating the other day. The local park near our house builds an ice rink for the winter. Jordan and Andrew always find a local rink or build their own at Andrew's house, as they are avid skaters and hockey players. So when I got home from the hospital, one of the first things they did was load me into the car with my wheelchair and drive over to the park. They strapped on their skates, got me into my chair and skated me around the ice. It was exhilarating, terrifying, and the most fun I have had in a while. Of course they also dumped me out of my chair and stole it to push each other around but that is to be expected with them.

Today is another fun day; it is the day of my half-birthday party. My mom and Jordan have decided to throw me a half-birthday party. I really do not grasp the concept of birthdays, aging, and time, so this is one way to show me. It is planned to be like a typical kids birthday party. I have learned there are themes, costumes, decorations, candy, food and games at this sort of thing.

I had a lot of trouble choosing a theme. There are too many to choose from: construction, tractors, dinosaurs, sports, colours, and the list goes on. Eventually after my family forced me to not have a construction, tractor, rainbow, dinosaur, first-responders themed party, I narrowed my theme down to just dinosaurs.

It is funny, one of the words that I often yell out like I do with 'fucking dingo', is pterodactyl. So a dinosaur theme seems fitting.

Andrew and Chris have just arrived to help Jordan, Mom and I set up for the party.

"Here Jenna, put this on. I got it for you," Jordan says as they hand me a dinosaur shirt. Everyone has been asked to wear a costume to the party and of course Jordan and I have matching pterodactyl shirts.

I gladly put it on and start looking at all the decorations. Andrew, Chris and Jordan put most of them up while I observe, feeling amused at the scene. This concept is wild and funny to me but I am grateful for the experience.

After setup is done, my party guests start showing up. The girls come in matching dinosaur onesies, Ron, Ellen and their kids come, my uncle Mark and Marie come with dinosaur gifts for me, Tresa from work, Uncle Ken and Aunt Sandi, and even my friend Emma facetimes to say hi. We all put our dinosaur party hats on and the party begins.

We start by doing a craft. We glue together these little gift bags that can be used to take home candy. They are designed like a dinosaur body and everyone can choose a face, tail and arms to glue onto their bag. When we finish with the candy bags my mom says, "It's time for a game! We are going to play pin the tail on the dinosaur. One at a time you come up and get a tail that has tape on it. You will be blindfolded and spun around three times and then have to find the dinosaur and guess where to pin the tail."

I ask if someone can go first to show me. My uncle Mark volunteers. I watch my mom blindfold her 'twin,' spin him around about ten times, and then gently push him in the direction of the dinosaur. He blindly stumbles forward and places his tail on the wall near the dinosaur's head. We all laugh with amusement as he makes a joke about being too old to be spun like that.

Next it is my turn. However, as we have learned in my physiotherapy, I have been labelled as a fall risk and have no balance skills. So closing my eyes makes me fall over. Therefore Jordan and Bella each stand on one side of me, supporting me. My mom puts the blindfold over my eyes and I lean into Bella on my left as she keeps me from falling. They help me stumble forward towards the wall, electing to not spin me around. I very slowly reach my left arm up towards the wall and place the tail on the dinosaur. I get it near his feet as that's as far as my tired arm will raise. Everyone cheers and I take the blindfold off. I smile with joy.

All the other guests take their turn at placing the tail on the dinosaur. Julia wins at the end and we all cheer for her.

Then we move on to other party games. We play musical chairs, which Heather wins, wink- murderer, and finish the games with a pinata. I love the concept of a pinata, as it is so fun to watch candy spread across the floor. It is hilarious watching all the adults run to the floor and scramble to fill their candy bags.

Once the candy is all claimed, Jordan says there is one more surprise. They go upstairs and come back a minute later. As they come downstairs the lights go off, and I become very confused. Jordan comes into view holding a cake with these sticks of fire coming out of it. Everyone begins singing Happy Birthday. I feel awkward and unsure of what to do. Everyone watches me as Jordan approaches. When they finish singing their song, my mom tells me to make a wish and blow out the candles. Bella chimes in by explaining the fire sticks are candles, and people blow them out and make a birthday wish to bring good luck to the next year of their life.

I start laughing at this crazy idea. Even though it seems so silly, I start to think of a wish. In my head I wish for everyone around me to be happy after supporting me so much. I take a deep breath in and blow out the candles. Everyone cheers and the lights flick back on.

"I didn't like when you were singing, I didn't know what to do." I say as everyone laughs.

"Some people love that moment and some don't. It kinda depends on if you like the attention on you," Ellen explains. I nod with understanding.

Jordan takes the cake upstairs and cuts it. They bring it downstairs again on dinosaur plates and start handing it out. When everyone has cake, Jordan approaches me. "Hey Jenna," they say and I turn and look at them. They smash of piece of cake into my face. Everyone starts laughing. I quickly grow angry and upset. Tears start to well up in my eyes. "Why did you do that?" I ask angrily.

"It's a thing people do at birthdays, it's like a prank," Jordan says.

The room feels slightly uncomfortable with me being upset. I try to hold my anger together and not have a meltdown. Most people haven't seen the emotional issues that I have, and it's embarrassing.

My mom quickly jumps in and brings me upstairs with Bella to clean off my face.

When I return downstairs there is an uncomfortable feeling in the air, as people don't know what to say.

My Aunt Sandi chimes in. "Alright make a note, no singing or putting cake in Jenna's face from now on. But let's keep partying."

That is enough to break the tension, conversations start up again and people move on from my small outburst. Jordan apologizes and I just feel grateful I didn't have a full breakdown in front of all these people.

The rest of the party continues smoothly with people chatting and laughing. As I start to get tired, people slowly start to leave. Once they are all gone, my mom helps me get upstairs. I get ready for bed as Jordan, Andrew and Mom clean up downstairs. Once I climb into bed I am very quick to fall asleep.

Chapter 12

March 2022

It is my 6th day back in the hospital. I had a relapse in my symptoms. Last week I was doing some schoolwork when my vision went weird and I got an intense headache. I tried to relax and see if sleep would help. However, over the next few hours, I started to lose feeling and functioning in my left side again. My speech got really stuttered but my memory remained. My roommate Julia brought me to the hospital, where they ran me through the stroke procedure. This time, however, they believed me. I was admitted again due to needing monitoring and an MRI scan which couldn't be done the same day. I have gotten my MRI which showed lesions again. My team of doctors still have no reason or understanding of what is happening. Rehab is the only answer at this point. The problem is there are no beds available on the rehab floor as there is a covid outbreak. So I remain on a general floor with about 10 minutes of rehab a day if I am lucky. Mom and I have been doing our own rehab work to get me home.

My mom walks into my room with a coffee for me. She sets it down on my table and turns to look at me. "What's going on? What is that face for?" she asks.

"Mom, I did it!" I exclaim.

"Did what, did you walk?" she asks with anticipation.

"No, but that would be cool. I got into the Master's program! I'm going to Trent," I say, my eyes filling with tears.

My mom grabs me into a hug with the biggest smile on her face. "Jen, I knew you could. No doubt in my mind. Look at you go, you applied last time from the hospital and here you are again getting accepted. I think this means you had to come back. But now never again!" my mom jokes.

I have gotten two prior rejections. One from the University of Toronto for their clinical psychology program and one from Ontario Tech University for their forensic psychology program. I have been feeling sad but also understand. My grades have dropped slightly this past year and my applications were probably not as good as they could have been, given the circumstances. I had begun to have serious doubts about being able to get into a Master's program, but that has all changed today. I am wanted, and I will go to Trent and kill it.

Back in December, I didn't even know what a Master's of Psychology was. My team had to explain it to me so I could finish my applications and submit them. I had no idea at the time what I was applying to, or if I even wanted to apply since I couldn't understand it, let alone walk. But as I learned things again, as I started school again, I knew that I had made the right choice to apply. Psychology is my passion, and I am so excited about this new journey.

My mom and I celebrate the occasion by drinking our coffees and chatting. We discuss life outside the hospital, and all the excitement occurring at home. When I finish my coffee I do some simple rehab exercises in my room. I work my arm till exhaustion and try to do some leg and ab exercises on my bed.

My mom and I begin to discuss coming home. "I feel like you should talk to the doctor about how long it will be until you get a bed on the rehab floor. We are just doing our own physio so what is the point in being here?" my mom explains. I agree but I also start getting upset at it all. It is all so frustrating and confusing. The doctors have said this could be my life from now on. My mom sees me getting upset. "Okay, enough about that. Let's go outside. Julia and Bella are coming by. Let's go meet them."

The weather has been exceptionally warm for March (or so I am told). Therefore I have been soaking up all the warmth and sunshine that I can this past week.

I wheel myself outside and see the girls. They brought me a tea as they always do. I tell them my news and they jump with excitement.

"Dude, we are so proud of you. Always knew you would get in. You literally are made for this," Bella says, and Julia agrees.

After our celebratory moment, we take a bit to just catch up on life together. I ask them to tell me about their life as I am tired of my own.

As we are talking I hear someone ask, "Is that Jenna?" I turn and look toward the voice.

"Oh wow! Hi!" I say.

It's Rachel, patient J's wife from the stroke floor.

I found her like a friend from my time on the floor in December. Each day she would see me in rehab and cheer me on, amazed with my progress. Her husband had been on the floor for a while before I got there. He was a younger man who had suffered a severe stroke but appeared to have major perseverance. I was always impressed when I saw him working in the gym.

Rachel and I start chatting about my relapse and me being back here. She tells me that her husband is still on the floor but they are sending him home soon as their time has come to leave.

It is heartbreaking to hear. Their life will never be the same. It's the same with my old roommate Paul. He is being sent home soon as well. Their families are now their caregivers, and it will never be the same.

Rachel turns to me and says, "This is horrible to say, but just remember you had the good kind of stroke. You are young. You can recover and you will. I've watched you. My husband, J, he won't ever be the same. I get about one sentence a day that he will understand. How do I choose my life in one sentence a day? How do I take him home and work to provide for us when he needs 24-hour care? You had the good stroke."

It isn't horrible to say, it is true. And us who have experienced this, who have witnessed the state of people on the rehab floor, know it's true. I did have the good kind of stroke. I am lucky as hell. I will recover to a point; I won't ever be the same again but for now at least, I am able to mostly take care of myself, I am able to communicate, I am able to re-learn the world. I did have the good stroke.

My heart breaks as we continue to talk to Rachel but I also feel ignited with perseverance like never before as she tells me J's whole story. How even he hasn't given up yet.

She also tells us that the whole floor is on lockdown due to covid and that it doesn't appear to be clearing up anytime soon. My mom and I discuss this as a further reason to discharge myself.

After quite a while, Rachel says she has to run. She commutes back and forth from her house in Havelock and she wants to get home before it's too late. I thank her deeply for talking with me, and for bringing me a feeling of familiarity in this place. I didn't even realize how badly I had missed her and all my other supports from the A2 floor until today.

Once Rachel leaves, I say goodbye to Bella and Julia as it's dinner time. My mom wheels me back inside. Once in my room, I transfer to my bed and my dinner arrives. Mom and I chat while I eat. "I think I want to ask to go home. Being here is pointless. They aren't doing anything, there is no rehab staff to work with me. I want to go home if I'm not getting a bed on A2 for a while," I say.

My mom agrees that it is the right decision. She tells me to discuss it with the doctors tomorrow. She packs her stuff up and says goodbye, needing to get home for dinner with Jordan. I say my goodbyes and she leaves.

I throw on Netflix and get cozy in my bed. A strong feeling of sadness washes over me. I just want to be home now that I've made up my mind. I don't want to be here anymore, alone. It's heartbreaking.

* * *

In the morning, after much discussion, my doctors agree that I can go home tomorrow. That it probably is the best choice since I already have access to outpatient rehab, and I have all my exercises I can do at home with support. Tomorrow can't come soon enough. I want out of here so badly.

All day I try to distract myself. I officially accept my offer to Trent University. I work on my thesis and I watch Netflix. The day drones on but I get through it. In the evening I pack all my stuff up, ready to go in the morning. I'm getting discharged around 11:00 am and I plan to be out of here by 11:01 am.

Finally, it is bedtime and I can sleep away the hours until home. I have a restless and impatient night of sleep.

In the morning I feel tired but happy. I get to leave today. Back to my life, back to good food, my family, my friends, and normalcy. It seems like the morning drags on forever, but finally the nurse brings me my discharge papers. I sign them quickly and give them back. They remove my IV and say I am good to go. My mom shows up as this is happening. She always has perfect timing.

She grabs my backpack and I transfer to my wheelchair and off we roll. This time no clap out, no big goodbyes to my support team. Just the two of us heading out to the car. A quiet goodbye with pleads that we don't have to do this again.

Chapter 13

April 2022

I click send as I submit my thesis to the department of psychology. I get the notification that my email has sent.

My undergraduate degree is officially accomplished. My thesis is submitted, my courses and exams are completed. I am done.

It has been a busy few weeks since being discharged from the hospital in March. I moved back into my house in Peterborough, as it is actually easier for me to be there and for the girls to get me back and forth to campus than to be living at home with my mom. I love living with them again. We have fun but they also respect my limits. They have started taking me to do things such as to the mind-blowing experience of Costco. And even places such as the bar or to play pool.

Bella and I have a weekly tradition of going to trivia at a local bar. She is amazing for taking me, having a blast, and then knowing when it is time to get me home. If I start looking like I have a headache (even though I refuse to say anything), or if I start screaming that people are fucking dingos or clicking my tongue too much, then she brings me home with no complaints. We often have a good group of people come with us. We invite all our friends and most come weekly, such as Connor, Jordan, and Andrew. But some weeks it is just the two of us. Either way, we have a blast and I love going.

Besides just taking me places, the girls have been showing me parts of the world I had no idea existed. We have weekly lessons where they drag out our whiteboard and explain concepts to me that I don't understand. They expose me to new TV shows and movies that are classics for our time. I love learning and they love exploring with me.

I also made a goal list with my mom. Before I came back to Peterborough I became quite unsure of myself. I have struggled with what my life has become, and who I am. I have become focused on trying to find myself, find who everyone knows me as, who I used to be before my brain injury, when really I need to work on creating myself.

In an effort to show me how amazing I am, my mom and I sat down and wrote a huge list of my goals. Big ones that I have, little ones, and even ones I have already accomplished. My mom wrote it down, as writing can still be a struggle for me. Then she taped the list in our living room. Each day she encourages me to read over my goals, cross off the ones I have achieved, and reflect on where I have come and where I am going. At first, I found this stupid, but I grew to love my goals list. I love seeing what I have done. I love having the visual of all I have achieved but also all that I plan to (and will) achieve, still to come.

So today, I cross 'finish my undergraduate degree' off the list. Another day, another goal achieved. I spend a few minutes staring at the list. I have already crossed off many goals, such as walk with no assistance, get accepted into a Master's program, cook a meal, learn to do laundry, and move back to my house in Peterborough. However, there are still so many to work towards, such as gain better filter skills, walk Addie down the aisle, learn the alphabet, and learn how to run. I feel gratitude in seeing what I have achieved but also passion as I add more goals to the list.

As I look at the goals still to achieve, I realize that I may be able to cross another one off this afternoon. I have physiotherapy this afternoon, and Blake had discussed us running this week. It makes me excited but also terrified.

I have come so far since starting my outpatient physiotherapy. I have been able to switch to a different brace on my left leg. I had been wearing an ankle-foot orthotic (AFO) but now am only using a simple ankle brace. My ankle is still very weak and easy to roll, so the brace stops that from happening.

I also have gained back some balance skills. During my original assessment for the outpatient program, I did a balance test. On this test, you receive a score out of 28. I scored a 15. It was explained to me that, on average, most seniors score a 26 out of 28 so my 15 is not ideal. It labelled me as a fall risk, and also gave my family a free pass to laugh at me (which they really don't need a free pass for, but at least they had an excuse). Currently, my balance still sucks, but it has improved a lot with my hard work. I practice standing on one leg for periods of time. I can actually stand on my right foot now, and keep my left one off the ground for over a minute! I still struggle standing on my left foot, standing on uneven ground, or closing my eyes while standing, but it will all come in due time.

* * *

Julia and I roll up to the hospital. I always bring my wheelchair to therapy because it allows me to sit if I am tired, but also it is the only way someone is allowed to come in with me. With covid protocols still in place, only essential caregivers are allowed to attend appointments with patients. As I appear a young healthy woman on the outside, if you don't look for the signs of my injury, then it is assumed I don't need a caregiver. Rather than continuing to get stopped and questioned about why someone is with me, I go in my wheelchair so no one bothers me. It makes me quite sad that this is my reality but I do what I have to do.

I still am not driving, I still get extremely tired after physiotherapy, and I still need someone with me to remember things I am told, such as my at-home exercises for the week. If someone is not with me, it makes it extremely difficult to get through an appointment. I make the therapist or doctor, or whoever, speak very slowly so I can write down every sentence they say. Then I get them to read it over and correct anything I have miswritten or misspelled and ensure I have all the information. It turns a ten-minute appointment into an hour. So I elect to use my wheelchair to make things easier, to not be hassled, and to not have to explain my situation every time I go somewhere.

Coming to physiotherapy has become quite routine for Julia and me, as it fits best with her schedule. We get through the screeners at the front doors of the hospital with her pushing me through. We clear the covid protocol and then I go and check in. I get my armband and off we roll to the elevators.

Once we get to the elevators today, I turn to Julia and say, "Do you think I will run today? What if I'm not ready?"

Julia smiles. "Bud you were born ready for this, let's make it happen." I smile and nod, knowing she is right.

I roll to the waiting area. Blake smiles at me through the window as he sees me roll up. The rehab assistant comes out and greets us. I roll myself into the rehab room and unbuckle my chair. I stand up and walk over to the bike machine to start my half-hour warmup and muscle-building. I start with ten minutes on the bike, then do leg curls and leg extensions, and then finish with five minutes on the arm bike. The five minutes of arm biking seem like hours for my left arm but I always enjoy the burn, knowing it is working my muscles hard. After the first half-hour, the patient that I overlap with leaves and I get a half-hour of one-on-one physio with Blake.

Blake always starts by asking me when I'm going to ditch the wheelchair. I laugh and say soon. Then he turns to Julia. "You think she is ready to run today?" he asks.

"Yes! I want to see that!" Julia responds with great enthusiasm.

I smile but feel the nerves building. "Are you sure I'm ready?" I ask.

"I think you're ready. But will you ever think you'll be ready? Besides, you know that we are in our last weeks of the program, and one of your goals is to learn to run again. I wouldn't do this if I didn't think you could, so why not try before it's too late?" Blake says.

"Okay then let's do it," I respond.

The outpatient stroke physiotherapy program only lasts for 12 weeks. After 12 weeks, you are discharged from the program and left to find your own private physiotherapy if you want to continue in rehab. I am coming up on my 12 weeks, so it is time to try my last few goals.

"To start I want you to just walk back and forth across the room, just like you've done before," Blake says.

I begin walking back and forth, thinking of my form. I remember to keep my hip held in so I don't hip-hike or let it pop out to the side when I get tired. I try to remember to step onto my heel and roll through my toes as Blake taught me to last week. From learning to walk with the AFO brace on, I got into a habit of stepping directly flat onto my foot instead of making it a fluid motion. Therefore I have to practice stepping heel to toe.

"That looks great Jenna. Now just like we've done before I want you to walk a little faster," Blake says.

I begin to walk faster. My gait gets a little sloppier but it still passes Blake's standards. I do this for a minute.

"Okay now run," Blake says.

I dead stop and look at him like he is crazy. "But how?" I ask.

"Nope, go back to walking, don't stop this time," Blake orders.

I begin to walk again, slightly faster than normal. "Yes like that, now run. Don't think, just do it," Blake tells me.

So I do. I awkwardly try to move faster. It feels like the weirdest, awkwardest movement ever. I am curious if I look as stupid as I feel. It is like my limbs are just flying around and I'm not going anywhere.

I see Julia and Blake break out into huge smiles.

"Jenna that was amazing!" Blake exclaims. "We have work to do to make it more efficient but that was so good for your first time. You ran!" he says.

I smile. I guess I did just run. Another goal has been achieved.

Blake and I spend the rest of the session working on my form. He gets me to walk with high knees around the gym. Then while doing high knees, I increase my speed until I am at a jogging pace. From there we practice running some more around the gym. We also work on the treadmill, going from critiquing my walking form and slowly increasing my speed to a run.

"Today was great. You absolutely crushed it," Blake says. "I want you to continue with your normal exercises. But now we will add some new ones. Really practice that walking form we have been working on. Watch for flat feet walking and keeping that left hip tight to your body. Don't let it get tired and hip-hike or pop to the side. Also, practice running. It will feel weird but you just have to get used to it. Practice starting and stopping. The more you practice, the less you will have to think about it, just like with your walking. If you practice enough then next week we can work on running with distractions just like we do with your walking."

"Thank you so much for today," I say.

"Of course, take care of yourself this week and remember to bug her about her homework," he says with a wink at Julia.

I get my coat on and sit down in my chair exhausted. Julia grabs her stuff and we begin to leave.

"Oh and by the way Jenna..." Blake says as we are about to leave.

I turn to him. "Yes Blake?"

"If you can run, you can dance. Go dance, friend," he says with a huge smile. I roll out the door with a nod and the biggest smile on my face.

"Guess we have to go out dancing this weekend then," Julia says. And we did.

Chapter 14

May 2022

My phone starts ringing, and I answer it. "Hey Jordan, how's it going?" I say.

"Hey kid, I'm alright but I have a question for you," Jordan says

"Shoot," I respond.

"Would you play baseball with me this summer?" Jordan asks.

"Umm I don't know. I probably wouldn't be very good. And who's playing?" I ask.

"Well, me and my friends Mark and Andrew, and a girl I play hockey with are going to play. You will be fine, it will be a good learning experience for you. So what do you say? No overthinking," Jordan tells me.

"I mean maybe," I say.

"Good, 'cause I already signed you up, so you have to. I'll text you the details so you have them. I love you, bye kid," Jordan says as they hang up.

I laugh at the phone call. I guess I'm playing baseball this summer.

I push the nerves away and continue to get ready for work. I am going to do my first on-site shift since before my stroke. One of my many jobs is working at an after-school program. My roommate Julia also works there. We are both supply staff, but I have taken more of an administrative role since my stroke. Today I am going into a site for an actual on-the-floor shift to see how it goes. It's nice because Julia is going into shift with me as an extra staff. Therefore if I need to step away from the kids, I can just tell Julia I need a break and not have to worry about staff-to-children ratios being compromised.

I finish getting myself ready and head downstairs. I knock on Julia's door and see if she is ready. She is, so we grab our things and head to her car.

We spend our drive to work like we always do, discussing how life is, how our partners are, and how school and work is going. The car for us is always like a catch-up time, and I love it.

When we get to work I feel nervous but also excited. I like my job as far as I know, I like working with kids, but they also can be a lot on my head. This shift should be interesting.

* * *

Julia and I walk out to the car. My head is killing me. The filter skills, the activity, the management of the program, it is all too much. I feel taken aback at how much those three hours wiped me out. How exhausted I am. But now I know. I'm not ready to return to work fully yet. My head can't handle it.

I begin to think about how funny my brain injury is. I sometimes forget I have one. But then I do what is such a little thing for everyone else and it wipes me out. My mom told me I used to work every night after a full day of school with no problem. My routine was work. Such as in high school I would go to school for the day then head to work after school. I would spend my weekends doing overnight respite shifts until I had to go back to school on Monday. Today I took my morning really chill in preparation for my shift, and now I can barely form words to speak to Julia. Even though I don't remember life before, I still find it funny to know how much life can change for anyone.

Julia and I spend some time debriefing the shift on our ride home. Julia drives and works through my aphasia with me to get where I'm at. Partway home we just turn on music to listen to, because talking isn't working for me.

When we get home, I eat dinner quickly and then climb into bed. Completely exhausted but now knowing a new limit. I shall continue to work on the administrative side of things for a while yet; playing games with 30 kids is not yet my strong suit.

* * *

I still feel exhausted after working yesterday. But I drag myself out of bed to get ready. My mom will be here soon to take me to my neurologist appointment. It's my six-month follow-up, which is crazy to think about. Six months already.

My mom shows up just as I finish drinking my coffee. I quickly brush my teeth and we head out the door. I'm feeling nervous today, as I always worry that I'll have to advocate that everything is not in my head or advocate for the time I deserve. I'm glad my mom is with me so I don't have to do this alone.

We get to the hospital, check in, and then have a short wait until we see my neurologist.

The appointment starts with my neurologist asking how I've been doing.

We go over how I haven't had any major mast cell reactions in months. How I finished the stroke physiotherapy program and did great. How I only have to wear my ankle brace during mentally stimulating activities or during physical activity.

My neurologist is impressed with my overall report. She informs me that my most recent MRI shows that the lesions on my brain have not grown at all since the scans done in March. This is great news.

She then conducts a bunch of tests on me. My left side still has some weakness and loss of feeling. But I pass all the speech and basic cognition tests, such as naming objects. Overall, there is serious improvement since December and we are all happy with where I am at.

To end the appointment we discuss our next steps. "Sadly, there is a huge gap in help for people like you. I'm afraid there is nowhere around here that will help you with your cognitive issues, that I'm aware of at least. You don't meet the age requirements for any of the programs to help post-stroke because of how young you are. The only places I know that would help are rehab centres in Hamilton, and that's just not an option with you being in school and where you are in life. It's a serious issue, but I don't know how you and I can solve it," my neurologist explains. She and my mom discuss some things we can do at home. But I know it won't be enough, and it breaks my heart. I remind myself that I can't give up; I still could get my full functioning back.

The neurologist and I discuss this for a bit, as I've done my research on recovery. It seems like the first six months are when I am expected to have the most recovery, and from there it's very slow gains if any. She confirms it does really slow down as time goes on, but that doesn't mean I won't see any recovery. I hope this is true.

"As well, I know it's scary that we don't know what happened. I'm not ruling anything out. This could have been a stroke, it could be multiple sclerosis, or it could be a rare condition that I don't know about. The problem is, we truly don't know much about the brain. Unless there is a perfectly clear scan to show what has happened, we are only guessing. For all we know there could be microscopic disconnects between the neurons in your brain, we just don't know how the brain works truly. I wish I could help you more. I could do more tests but they won't confirm anything fully. Take a spinal tap for example. In 90% of people, there will be a specific inflammatory protein in their spinal fluid if they have MS. So if you have a positive spinal tap for the protein, then there's a good chance you have MS. But then I would also have to consider you have mast cell and arthritis; what if you were just in a flare and the inflammatory protein was there because of that? What if your results were negative; maybe you are just one of the 10% of people that don't have this protein with their MS condition. There is nothing else I can do to perfectly figure this out, and I don't want to do invasive tests if I can avoid them because your mast cell is balanced right now," she explains.

To me, this is the best outcome I could have hoped for besides a magical fix-everything diagnosis or pill.

I am reassured that I am not crazy, that I can't fake being paralyzed for months or losing my memories or speech, and I can't fake brain lesions or blown pupils even though the ER doctors said I was faking. My neurologist tells me she is on my team, she is here for me and not going anywhere. She will fight this fight with me.

But the only fight right now is to wait this out for a bit. We agree that if I need anything I will touch base with her. I will check in with my school to see if they have any cognitive resources she doesn't know about. And as long as things keep going smoothly as they are, then we will push my next routine brain and spine scans until a year, as things seem to be in remission for now.

My mom and I leave the office exhausted but grateful. It was probably the longest time a doctor has ever given me. I was there for over an hour. Over an hour of actually listening to me, wanting to help me, believing me.

That is the first appointment in a long time that my mom and I didn't walk out feeling crushed.

My mom has told me my history of fighting with doctors to figure out my mast cell and arthritis issues. It was over a two-year battle of being super sick. I lost tons of weight (and I'm very small to begin with), I was in constant pain and couldn't breathe half the time. But doctors assumed with my age I couldn't have arthritis, even though it was the only possible solution left to explore, and I couldn't have mast cell because it's so rare.

But when my rheumatologist saw me after waiting a year for a referral, she instantly said, "No question you have rheumatoid arthritis and you need a new allergist, stat, to figure out your skin and allergy issues. This is brutal."

My allergist in Peterborough kept trying to get me into a different allergist who specialized in mast cell disorder based out of Toronto. However, after four different requisitions being sent I finally was told he didn't have time as he was dealing with people reacting to the Covid vaccines.

It took me being admitted to the hospital for a week with an out-of-control anaphylaxis reaction, and having my 'second mom' Leisa send me allergist information, to finally get somewhere. I called and begged allergists to see me. Finally, one in Kingston believed me. She told me, “I don’t even care what you have; you are 19 years old in a hospital bed from this. Call me as soon as you get discharged and we will get you here to Kingston for testing and to start a new med plan to get you stable.”

She is the one still following me today. The one who has gotten me stable by starting me on five different medications back in 2020, and together we’ve been able to work it down to one daily med plus monthly Xolair injections.

So today, walking out of the neurologist appointment, it is a relief. My stroke makes my daily life very different, and often difficult for me. But my neurologist doesn’t. She believes me; she is fighting for me and with me. And that is the greatest relief my mom and I could have today.

* * *

I have come home from my appointment and crushed a nap. Now Julia, Heather and I are sitting on our kitchen floor as we often do, just hanging out and talking. Our kitchen floor always seems to be the gathering space, as uncomfortable as it is. I had just finished telling the girls about how my appointment went and how relieved I am, even though we have no answers.

“So how are you feeling now that you’ve slept? I know you were exhausted, but how is your head now?” Julia asks me.

"It actually feels good. I passed out hard for a while and I feel rested, which is nice for a little bit at least," I reply.

Julia's face brakes out into a smile as she grins at Heather. Julia gets up. "Go throw your shoes on Jenna, I got a surprise for you," she says.

"You want to come?" Julia asks Heather.

"I'm okay, I don't like that smile, I think I'll stay here," Heather says while laughing.

I put my shoes on as Julia puts hers on. She grabs my car keys. "Let's go, we will give your car a run," Julia says.

I go outside and jump in the passenger seat while Julia gets behind the wheel. She backs out of the driveway and starts driving across town. We chat about her day as we head over to the east side of town.

Julia pulls into a parking lot.

"Hey, this is where we went swimming," I say with excitement.

The other day, Julia and I had come to the park to work out outside. We had done a workout and then she had brought me down to the little beach to feel what the sand is like. I loved feeling the sand, and its warmth on my feet. I was feeling the sand run through my fingers while watching a mom and son swim through the water. They appeared to be the only ones brave enough to go in the cold water.

Everyone else was enjoying the May weather by suntanning on the beach, knowing the water was still cold. Julia had stood beside me and said that one day we could come back and go swimming. I smiled up at her and said, "I'll go in if you go in." She laughed and asked if I was serious. I stood up and took off my shirt. She started laughing and took off hers. We stood on the beach in our shorts and sports bras, laughing. She told me to wait a minute and she set up her phone to record.

"Just remember don't go deep and then you can still stand. And close your mouth, it's like the shower kinda, you don't want to drink the water or choke," Julia explained as I nodded, nervous but also filled with exhilaration.

Julia grabbed my hand and we started running together towards the water. We ran in and when it got up to our waists she told me to jump. Hand in hand we jumped in the water and stood up laughing. It was like a movie. Everyone on the beach disappeared as I had this unreal sensation of the water around me. Julia showed me how to blow bubbles while putting my head under, she showed me how to splash water at others and how to love being in the water. That day was pure joy.

I snapped out my swimming memory as Julia got out of the car. I followed her around to the front of my car.

"You still feel good?" she asks me.

"Yes, but will you tell me why please?" I say laughing.

She holds up my keys. "I'm going to teach you to drive again."

My face lights up and I burst out laughing. "No fucking way," I say.

"Bud, I wouldn't do it if you weren't ready. You cleared your six-month follow-up. It's time," Julia says.

I shake my head while laughing, but I take my keys out of her hand and go to the driver's seat. I sit down and take a minute to just sit. I put my hands on the steering wheel and see what it feels like. I put my right foot on the brake pedal, then move it to the gas.

Julia starts with basic instructions. She has been talking me through what she is doing while she has driven recently, to get me thinking about it. We go over the basics again.

"It's time. If you feel up to it, then let's do this. Just start with some laps around the parking lot," Julia says.

So I do. I do laps, I practice driving, breaking, signalling, and steering. I feel comfortable; it's natural.

"Julia, it's there. I don't remember driving but it feels natural," I say with excitement.

We practice parking, more of the basics, and Julia yells commands at me to test my reflexes a bit. I perfect each motion. After a while, Julia tells me to go to the road. "It's quiet around here, it's mid-day before school is out. Not many people will be on the roads and we will stay on all the country roads. If you get tired at all then say so and we will stop, but otherwise let's drive bud," Julia says.

So I turn onto the road and I drive. I drive, not wanting to stop. I feel free again. But I also feel a headache coming on and I know I have to stop. I still need to be gentle with my brain. I pull over and Julia drives us back to our house.

When I get out of the car I laugh with my restored freedom. I know I'm not ready to just jump in the car by myself or drive for long periods of time. But I am on the path to having my freedom back, to being more independent, and to checking another goal off my list. And holy shit, it feels unbelievable.

Chapter 15

June 2022

Mom and Jordan have come to go for a walk with me. A few weeks prior the girls and Bella's boyfriend Mike had taken me to the Peterborough Zoo. I had fallen in love with it. We had gone a few times in my wheelchair so I could get used to the atmosphere. But today, Jordan and Mom are taking me without my chair. I am challenging myself to get out more without my chair when I know the circumstances. To push my brain more to see what the limits are. And so far today is going well.

We have made it all the way down to the camel exhibit. I think they are hilarious animals, so it is a nice rest to watch them for a while. My brain is actually doing quite well so we take a longer loop back to the start of the zoo.

"So the wedding is this weekend; you feel ready for it?" my mom asks.

The family I do respite work for and my second family, Leisa and Cameron (aka Mom and BBQ Dad), are getting married and I am a bridesmaid.

"Yeah, there isn't much to be ready for. I just have to put on the dress and show up," I say.

"Well yeah but you do have to do a bit more, like we always say you have to walk Addie down the aisle, you know," my mom replies.

"Well yeah, we always say that. But what does that mean?" I ask.

Jordan and my mom look at each other and burst out laughing. "Jenna do you know what happens at a wedding ceremony?" Jordan asks me.

"What do you mean ceremony? Like I thought I just showed up and they would be married and we would dance like you said," I reply.

"Well not exactly. There is a ceremony, where you will have to walk with Addie down the aisle in front of all the guests," my mom says.

I instantly start sweating. "What did you think the rehearsal dinner was for kid?" Jordan asks.

"Well, I thought it was weird but we had to rehearse how to eat and dance before the wedding," I say.

Again Jordan and my mom crack up with laughter and I join them as I realize this is way different than what I thought it would be.

So in the middle of the Peterborough Zoo, with tons of people around, staring at us like we are crazy, Jordan and my mom shamelessly show me a demonstration of what a wedding ceremony is. They show me how there is an order that people walk in, how I will walk with Addie up and back down the aisle, how I will have to stand at the front of the ceremony until it is over.

When they explain that Leisa and Cam will have to kiss to seal the deal, I burst out laughing. "That's the weirdest thing. Everyone is just cheering as your stick your tongues down each other's throat," I say laughing. Jordan and Mom laugh with me.

"Well not exactly, but you do kiss, it's like a sign of love and stuff," my mom says.

"If I ever get married, I'm electing for like a crisp high five and then we can kiss later," I say, laughing.

"I'll let Pat know you're down for a crisp high-five," my mom says with tears in her eyes from laughing so hard.

"This whole rehearsal dinner makes so much more sense now," I say. "I didn't realize I actually had to do stuff. I feel scared cause I'll probably screw it up."

"Yeah you just might, but you know how cute Addie is, so no one will even be looking at you," Jordan says with a smile. "Plus, I'll be there and Mom will be there. We are there to help you if you need it. Just remember how much you love Leisa and Cam, and how happy you are for them. They aren't going to be mad if you screw up. You will so be fine," Jordan says.

And I was.

* * *

I was drunk and happy. I was dancing with Addie and Leisa, absolutely overjoyed. I had made it through the rehearsal dinner. I had made it down the aisle without falling. At the last minute I panicked and decided not to wear my heels. Leisa didn't care what I wore, she just cared that I was there. And I'm glad I made the decision; it made it seamless. Addie wasn't thrilled at first to walk with me down the aisle. She wanted her tablet and wheelchair, but I grabbed her hand and guided her forwards as she tried to go back to her chair. I pointed forward and said "Ads, look," and as soon as she saw all the people and her dad waiting at the end of the aisle, she grinned and off we went walking effortlessly together. We both made it through the ceremony and I even held in my laughter when Mom and BBQ Dad kissed (which was hard as my mom made eye contact with me from the crowd and laughed). Addie didn't want to come out of her wheelchair so I pushed her down the aisle as she rocked and laughed with excitement.

I had made it through pictures and dinner with no issues. I had overcome my own awkward moments as I re-met so many of my friends and family who I had no recollection of. Mom and BBQ Dad succeeded in making me cry with their speech. I even overcame my speech confidence and told a story to the room of how I met Mom and BBQ Dad with Cassandra, to get the bride and groom to kiss (I'll never forget your dance skills, BBQ Dad - haha).

I had completed my responsibilities and done it effortlessly. So now was my dancing and happy time. Time to chill, time to celebrate the day and the nerves being gone. And it was the best night I could have imagined for my BBQ parents. I love them so deeply.

* * *

I still don't want to go today. But my people want me to go. They find it important even though I don't understand the point of it. However, Julia and I agreed that we would suffer through it together at least.

Last night in a panic I decided on my grey dress for the occasion. Julia now zips it up for me. I put on my ankle brace and clasp my heels over top.

I look in the mirror and give myself a hesitant smile. I remind myself that I can do this. That it will be okay.

Julia and I climb into the car. She drives us to campus. To our graduation ceremony.

My mom, Ellen, Heather, and Julia's family are meeting us there. Julia and I have to go early to get in the graduate line-up and such.

It is sheer panic when I get there. I'm singled out because of my wheelchair. I can't do the walk into the ceremony with the rest of the graduates because there are many sets of stairs. I have to choose between my chair and obviously being different, or walking and risking falling.

We agree that I will meet the group at the top of the bridge. It cuts out some of the walking and then it is only a flight of stairs down, a walk across the Bata podium and a flight of stairs up to my seat. The staff helping me agrees that I can walk in with Julia to help me up the stairs even though we aren't near each other in line. She sees the panic and tears and does her best to reassure me.

I get her to explain everything to Julia. They tell the person I'm sitting beside during the ceremony the plan so she can save me a seat.

The graduates start the walk out of the student centre, over to Lady Eaton College. The staff member wheels me over to the library and we take the elevator up to the top of the bridge. We wait there for the rest of the graduates. I get ready to walk. The graduates start walking by in their line and the staff pushes me in my place beside Julia.

When we get to the top of the stairs, we pause as everyone continues around us. I panic. "Stand up, I've got you bud," Julia says.

I take a huge breath and stand. I steady myself, grab Julia's arm with a death grip, and we walk down the stairs. The staff carries my wheelchair behind me. I walk across the podium towards the second set of stairs. We get to the stairs and I take a deep breath.

"You're good, we are almost there," Julia says to me.

We start going up the stairs one at a time slowly. I look to my right as someone holds out their hand. It's another graduate I've never seen before. "Let's do this together," she says. And she and Julia get me up the stairs. At the top I collapse down into my wheelchair and the staff pushes me over to the chair I will sit in with the other graduates.

I transfer to the chair and the staff goes over the plan with me. When it is my turn she will bring me my wheelchair back to sit in. The row of graduates I'm sitting with will get up, walk around the back of the stage and wait till it is each of our turns to walk across the front of the stage. She will bring my wheelchair so I can have it until it is my turn. I'm determined to walk, not wheel across the stage.

Once everything is in place I can breathe until it's my turn. I take a minute and turn to see who is around me. It turns out that Julia is in the row right in front of me. I also turn to my right, and it is the girl who helped me up the stairs. I smile at her and thank her.

"No problem, I'll help you get into place too. We've got this. Don't be nervous," she says with the warmest smile.

The rest of the ceremony drags on. It feels long as we sit in the scorching sun. The people around me make jokes about the drone Trent is using, and how loud it is. We graduates can't hear anything that is being said about us because of it. But then it is my row's turn to go across the stage. I'm near the end. I wait and the staff brings me my wheelchair. I transfer to it and they wheel me into place.

I get my picture taken by the photographer while I wait. My new friend is in front of me. She will go and I will be next. Right before she goes, she turns around and bends down to straighten out my gown. "You can do this. I'll see you back at our seats," she says with a smile.

I smile at her as she turns and walks across the stage.

I reach up and hand my name card to the MC. The staff squeezes my shoulder. I stand as they read my name and I begin to walk across the stage. I shake the hands of those giving out the degrees. I hear Julia scream for me. People clapping. I smile, I'm doing it.

I get across the stage to where the professors are sitting. My thesis supervisor gets up and shakes my hand with congratulations. My soon-to-be Master's supervisor gets up and hugs me. "Congratulations, you so deserve this," he says.

I finish walking and collapse into my wheelchair. I'm wheeled over to my seat. I congratulate the girl beside me just as they announce Julia's name. I cheer as loud as I can for her as she strides across the stage.

It feels like just as quickly as the panic had started, it's over as they wrap up the ceremony. Now all I have to do is walk back across the stairs and podium to the top of the bridge where my chair will be waiting for me again. When it's my turn, I stand. Julia slides in beside me on my left side and the girl beside me offers me her arm. I walk down the stairs with the two of them helping me. The rest of the graduates pass us as we slowly go down the stairs. But I don't care, I did it. I overcame the panic and I didn't fall. I walked across the stage like I said I would.

As much as I didn't want to come today, as much as I still don't understand the point of the ceremony with all these people I don't know, I'm still happy I came. It made my mom proud, I was reminded how amazing random strangers can be, and I took another step towards overcoming my fear of my disability and people judging me. It is a good day.

* * *

I looked up at Julia in awe. We were standing in the park with Andrew and Tyler. The town is lighting off fireworks to celebrate Beaumont days. Julia looks down at me and smiles seeing the joy on my face.

"Julia, if I text my mom to look outside can she see how pretty these are?" I ask. Julia starts laughing. "That was adorable but no. We are thousands of miles away from your mom. There is no way she could see them," Julia says.

"Oh okay," I say with disappointment.

"Look at the tree there," Julia says while pointing to a tree in front of us to the left. I look at the tree. "See how you can't see the fireworks as well through the tree, like it blocks them. Think of how many trees there are between here and your mom," Julia explains. I nod with understanding and try to live in the moment with the beautiful light show in front of me.

The past few days have been a whirlwind. Julia, Andrew, Jordan and I are in Alberta. We flew out here right after graduation on the 10th of June and are staying with family until the 19th.

Jordan and Andrew told me that we had a trip planned in April of 2020 to drive out here; however, with the pandemic we never got to do it.

When I was offered the chance to present at the Canadian Psychological Association Annual Conference in Calgary, we saw it as a chance to do the trip we always wanted to do. I had also invited Julia to come so I had someone to attend the conference with, and of course she was thrilled to come.

Over the past few days, I learned what an airport and airplane are (turns out it is not just a car that has wings attached to it and you need a pilot to fly it, not just Andrew), I re-met my family who lives in Edmonton, I learned what a parade was, I went to an Edmonton Oil Kings game, was blown away that there are time changes and different sun setting times, did some exploring, and now am amazed at fireworks.

Our next few days are also packed full of exploring. We have plans to go to Jasper, to visit the Edmonton mall, to watch the kid's soccer games, and eventually Julia and I will end up in Calgary for the conference next weekend. The week is filled with adventure and good times, not just for me but for everyone involved.

After the firework show is over, I wheel myself back to the car. We all pile in and make the short drive home. Once home, I get ready for bed. It is crazy that the sun has just set and it is already midnight. I climb into bed and fall asleep quickly, exhausted from the crazy past few days but excited for what else the week entails.

* * *

Julia and I are waiting for our coffee. We got up this morning, got ready for day three of the conference, and decided to take a walk to grab a coffee before my presentation. Once our coffee is ready, we walk over to the conference centre and get the technology set up with my thesis supervisor and other colleagues. Now we just have to wait till 9:00 am. I am the first presenter in this morning's symposium. Overall, I don't feel as nervous as I thought I would. More just wanting it to start.

Julia and I do a lap around the conference centre while we wait for the symposium to start. We reflect on our past few days. We had a blast this week. We had so many new experiences. I got to ride a rollercoaster for the first time that I can remember. We got to explore Jasper, which is now on my bucket list to go back to, when I can actually walk on uneven ground so we can explore more. Our van broke down in the middle of nowhere on our way back to Beaumont from British Columbia, leaving us stranded alone at 10:00 pm while we waited for Tyler to drive three hours to come pick us up. We got to explore the Calgary zoo with Jordan and Andrew before they drove back to Edmonton when dropping Julia and me off at the conference. We had a week full of fun and many firsts for me.

Today I will present, and then Jordan and Andrew will pick us up. We will drive back to Edmonton (while stopping at a Canyon) and later tonight we fly back to Ontario.

I just have to kill my presentation in the meantime.

Julia and I go back into the conference room. People are now starting to show up, and the nerves kick in. My colleagues reassure me that I will be fine. My supervisor goes over how the symposium will go, with him doing my introduction, then I'll present, followed by the other three presentations, and then we will have group question time.

9:00 am hits. Julia starts the facetime with my mom, Ellen and Pat back home so they can watch me present. My supervisor starts his introduction. "To start off our symposium, I have the honour of introducing my student, Jenna, who just completed her undergraduate thesis with me on this topic, and has continued to work with our research team on this project," he says.

I stand up and walk behind the podium. I give my supervisor a nod in thanks and start my presentation. "Thank you. As said, I am Jenna. I just completed my undergraduate degree while working on this project and will enter my Master's of Psychology in September. Before I begin I want to take a quick moment and just give everyone a disclaimer. Six months ago I had a stroke that has left me with some speech and aphasia issues. Therefore if I stutter please bear with me. Also if I start saying words that make no sense, please tell me because I want to be able to tell you our research and not have my aphasia confuse people. With that being said, let's get into it! I along with my colleagues have been evaluating quantitative experts' views of effect sizes in psychology..."

I finish my presentation effortlessly. I don't even remember getting through it all. The room fills with applause. I smile, collect my notes, and take my seat. For the rest of the symposium, I feel like I'm not in the room while I ride the high of presenting. Once the last talk finishes, I get through the question period with no stress. I was mostly worried about the questions and not being able to answer them, but I have no issues with what is asked, and my research team is there to back me up.

Once the questions are done, people begin filing out of the room. My research team congratulates me; they even say that they couldn't have done it better themselves, and they mean it. Julia congratulates me for killing it. I didn't even stutter or have aphasia.

In this moment, I remember how much I enjoy public speaking. How I am a natural at it. How I may struggle sometimes with my speech but how I haven't fully lost my power of speech. How I am gaining that power back as my confidence increases. Who knows, maybe a career in public speaking is where I'll end up. But for today, I am just over the moon with how well that went.

After talking with a few people who had questions or congratulations after the symposium, Julia and I pack up our stuff. We run into a few other Trent students from the conference, and I learn how big of a deal it is that I gave a talk. Everyone else did poster presentations, not symposium talks. Poster presentations are a big enough accomplishment, don't get me wrong, but the other students were shaken that I had the confidence to do a talk. It gave me even more confidence, and I learned how big of a deal these conferences are. I feel empowered.

Julia and I head back to our hotel room. We grab our stuff and check out. We sit on the curb for about ten minutes going over how amazing this trip is. Then Jordan and Andrew pull up in the van. We hop in and head back to Edmonton to get home.

That evening we have dinner, and then go to the local park to play a game of baseball with the kids before our flight. During the baseball game, we have some lost bets, and Andrew and I have to wear underwear outside of our clothes to the airport. I have to rock holey boxers, and Andrew wears a bright purple thong on the outside of his jeans. Needless to say, Andrew gets stopped and searched by security.

Our flight ends up delayed but eventually we get on, have a smooth flight, and make it back home by the next morning, where Pat picks us up from the airport. Four tired but blessed kids.

Alberta Baby was a trip that holds a special place in my heart. It was a one-of-a-kind trip, and I loved every second of it.

Chapter 16

July 2022

I have been continuing to work as a research assistant during the summer for my Master's supervisor. I have worked as an RA for him since the second year of my undergrad and he still keeps me around. This summer I have put in some part-time hours since I wanted to stay active in the lab, as I will be joining it in September. I am also working full-time for the YMCA, but I balance my hours between the two positions. It is helping me make up for lost income from December to May of this past year.

Recently I was in the lab running participants for my lab-mate, who is just finishing up her thesis. My lab-mate and I got talking about a conference she was going to attend in a couple of weeks in Halifax. She would be presenting her work, that I had helped collect data for. She mentioned that I should talk to our supervisor about going with her. So I did, and we all agreed that it would be good for me to go and for her to have someone from the lab go with her.

So here I am sitting back at the airport just a bit over a month since Alberta, waiting to fly to the other side of the country.

This trip is a lot different, however, as I am doing it alone in a sense. I am traveling with my lab-mate, who is probably the sweetest person I could travel with for this occasion. However, none of my core group of people are coming with me. And my wheelchair is being left at home.

I wanted to bring it with me, but it makes travelling a lot different. Someone has to help me with my bags, opening doors, ensuring the uber can fit my wheelchair, and so on and so on. So instead of putting that on my lab-mate, I have chosen to try this adventure without it.

We have just cleared security and are now waiting at our gate for boarding, enjoying a coffee together. I am counting the lines in the carpet and trying to zone into the task. I have a stroke headache coming on, and I'm worried about how it will affect this process. I know all I have left to do is to walk to the plane and find my seat, and then I have two hours to sleep this off. But that in-between of waiting and then having to walk and find my seat is making me very nervous. What if walking is too much and I limp or fall? What if I can't count the numbers properly and can't find my seat? What if I look dumb or start yelling out words at people? All the 'what ifs' are running through my head. So I count the lines on the carpet and breathe. I try to ignore everything around me; the noise, the colours, the movement. I try to zone into the carpet and subside the panic of not having my wheelchair.

My lab-mate taps my arm. "We can board now," she says with a reassuring smile.

I stand up shakily. I pick up my backpack and begin to walk. I watch my lab-mate show the flight attendant her ticket and ID, and I repeat the same motions. I walk down the gate to the plane. I begin to feel more confident. I'm almost there. I use the seats of the plane to steady myself as I walk the aisle and read the row numbers. I finally find mine. But then I panic. I have to get my carry-on into the compartment above my head. I try to pick it up with my left arm and I struggle; I know there is no way I can lift it above my head with only my right arm. I'm too short to do this with one arm.

I start sweating. I'm holding up the line. People need to get by me. I have to speak.

I turn to the man waiting behind me. "Could you maybe help with this, this, this." I have lost the word I need but I point to my bag and then point to the compartment. He gives me a bit of a strange look but nods and picks my bag up and places it in the compartment for me. I nod as a thank you and step into my row. I take my backpack off and slide it under the seat in front of me as I collapse into my own seat.

Almost instantly after take-off my eyes close and I fall into a deep sleep until the plane descending wakes me up. That wears me out but I did it.

* * *

The conference had gone smoothly. I loved being there, learning, networking and just being surrounded by like-minded people. My lab-mate presented like a natural! I also re-met an old friend who I knew from my days working camp in high school, and we grabbed a coffee together, both finding it hilarious to re-meet at a conference across the country. Our plane ride home was less daunting as the Halifax airport was less busy; still painful for my head, but a bit better. Pat picked me and my lab-mate up from the airport and drove us home. Overall it was a successful trip to Halifax.

As hard as that had been, it had proven to me that being a bit adventurous again was not a bad thing. Therefore my friend Bella and I have planned for me to go visit her for a weekend. She is living in Toronto for the summer as she is doing an internship there. I have wanted to visit this big city that everyone talks about, so we agreed that I would take the go-train down and spend a few days with her touring around.

Currently, I am sitting in the car in the train station parking lot. My mom drove me here and is waiting for me to be ready. I can see the train tracks from where we sit in the car. All I have to do is get out of the car and walk over there. But I feel like I can't move. The train I want to take is there, boarding. But I can't move. My mom looks at me and says, "Let's just watch this one and then you can take the next one. It won't be that long of a wait." I nod in agreement.

I finally get out of the car after a few more minutes of sitting. I lean against the car, feeling panicked. After a few minutes the train starts to pull away. I stare after it, amazed at how it works. I've never seen anything like it.

I pull out my phone and text Bella that I didn't make the train. That I'll catch the next one. Of course she is fine with this.

I am partly panicked because I have decided to not take my wheelchair as I've been told Toronto is really busy. My mom thinks it will be hard for me to get around Toronto in my wheelchair so she told me to not take it. Bella is indifferent and will work with whatever I decide. I figure if I could survive the airport, then I can survive a weekend without my wheelchair, even if that means Bella and I can't do everything we want to do because my head hurts.

I stand in the parking lot for a while, just soaking in the environment and talking myself back into doing this.

I'm beginning to find ways to help myself in new environments. For example, I find comfort in going places early to get used to the surroundings before I become immersed in them. When we went to the airport to go to Alberta, the gang sat with me out front for a few minutes and waited for me to be ready to go inside. Then when we got inside, they refused to check in until I was ready. We just sat in the hustle and bustle for a while until I could move. Or when I go to a restaurant, I pick my seat strategically to either sit with a wall to one side of me to block out some noise, or I pick the seat that will have the least visual stimulation to reduce my headache. It is comforting to do these things. They help my head.

The next train is set to arrive in a few short minutes. My mom grabs my arm. "Jenna, you can do this. Let's go. I will walk you right up to the door of the train," she says.

With my mom's help, I pick up my bags and start to walk towards the train platform. We get to the platform, and I stare up at how tall the train is. I'm amazed that there are two layers to it. People can sit on the second story of it. Wild!

My mom brings me to the accessibility cart. I stare at the train for a few minutes until someone asks me, "Can I help you?" It is a man in a uniform. He explains that he is the customer accessibility guide and will be riding in the cart I'm standing in front of. My mom asks me if she can tell him my situation. I agree. She explains that I have a brain injury and have no memory of travel like this, but that I'm going to ride the train to Toronto to visit my friend.

The man turns to me and tells me his name is Bryan. He asks what my name is, and I tell him. "Well Jenna, I will be your friend on this train. You come here, sit right there. I will tell you when your stop is coming up. I will tell you what platform we are going to stop at Union Station on, and then I'll make sure you text your friend the platform so they can meet you right outside the accessibility cart. And this train will not leave that platform until I see you with your friend. You are going to be okay, and we will do this together," Bryan says as he points me to a seat. Tears well up in my eyes. I hug my mom and say goodbye, feeling more confident about this. I take a deep breath, look up and down the platform at the train once more, and walk up the ramp to my seat.

Bryan and I have a great ride together. We chat about his job, we chat about my stroke, and we chat about each station we stop at.

We start approaching Union Station, and Bryan tells me to text Bella that we are arriving on platform 7. Bella tells me she is there waiting.

After a few minutes we pull up to Union Station, and Bryan tells me this is my stop. I pick up my bags and start to head off the train while thanking Bryan. He stops me. "I just want you to know I think your story is amazing. You so got this. Keep going and always looking ahead. Thank you for sharing your story with me," he says.

"Thank you so much," I reply. "I really appreciate everything you have done this train ride for me. You really made this so much smoother."

We smile at each other and then I turn and walk off the train. I see Bella standing right outside the platform. I walk quickly to her, and she grabs me into a huge hug. "You did it! You made it!" she says. Tears well up in my eyes as I agree with her; I did do it. We hug tightly until the train starts to pull away. I let go of Bella with my right hand and wave goodbye to Bryan. Another stranger who will always mean something to me.

Bella and I then make the adventure to her house. We start by walking to the subway. The subway blows my mind. Bella carries my bags and holds my hand as we get on and find a seat. I know I have to move quickly as the subway won't wait for me, but it is blowing my mind to see and experience. After the subway, Bella explains that we could walk to her house, but it's about 20 minutes and I've already had a lot put on my head tonight. So we agree to take a bus. The third new transportation method that I find mind-blowing. We get through the bus ride without any major issues, just more of a lack of understanding for me. After the bus, we take a short minute walk to Bella's house. It is also mind-blowing to see a neighbourhood like this. So nice and so different than my home in Peterborough. Once inside I take a few minutes to look around. Bella brings me down to her room. We get ready for bed and I quickly fall asleep, exhausted from my adventures.

* * *

The rest of my weekend in Toronto was amazing. Bella and I saw some staple tourist things such as the CN tour, we walked into the Eaton Centre shopping mall (and walked out again as it was an instant headache), we walked by the Roger's Centre and the aquarium. We drank paper planes and ate fancy food that you can't find in Peterborough. But the best part of it was spending time with Bella, just being us and having fun, but also the transportation. The transportation blew my mind; I had no recollection of methods such as the subway, and they are amazing.

I don't want to share all the details of our weekend because it was special to us. It was a new experience for me, and a growing experience for our friendship. We truly learned the balance between exploring and me being okay. Bella was amazing at knowing when I needed a break but also giving me all the fun we could handle. And I am so glad I did it.

* * *

When I first had my stroke, the people closest to me in my life knew about it but otherwise I didn't really tell anyone. However, when my isolation story was made public and on the news, obviously a lot of people who knew me ended up finding out about my story.

When people found out, they reached out. My old dance teacher was one of many who reached out to my mom.

It turns out I used to be a competitive dancer. I danced from I was four years old until I went off to university. I was at Hype Danz studio in Courtice for many, many years and Margarita, the owner of the studio, was my all-time favourite dance teacher because of her positivity and inclusivity.

So when she found out about my memory loss and situation, she told my mom that as soon as I was able to go, I had to go and tour the studio to see if I remembered anything.

Today is that day.

My mom and I are just arriving. I stand outside the studio for a minute, staring at the door. It is new to me; I don't remember it. I have that small disappointing feeling creeping back in that I get whenever the memories don't come back, but I push it away. I'm not even inside the building yet; there is still a chance.

I take a deep breath as I always do, and head to the door. We go inside and instantly Margarita welcomes me with the sweetest hello.

Her two kids are also there and they say hello, but sadly I have no memory of them.

Margarita starts with a tour of the studio, showing me all the rooms and the pictures. She and my mom also discuss the old studio layout to see if I can remember it. As much as I grew with this studio, the studio also grew while I was there. I started dancing with Hype when it was in a renovated barn and now it is located in a more upscale location.

I do not have any recollection of the studio in my mind. However, Margarita gets an idea. "I have old competition videos of you. Maybe those would help," she says. We spend the next while watching me on stage competing. It's crazy to see that person, me, moving so elegantly compared to how I move now. How I am there running and jumping and flipping, just dancing all over the stage when six months ago I couldn't move half my body.

That person on that stage is thriving; I was thriving, I guess. This studio was my second home, my therapy through the trauma with my uncle, my therapy through my dad abandoning me, and my therapy through my shitty high school years. This was me thriving and I want to thrive like that again.

Margarita emails me copies of all the videos. Then she turns to me and asks, "Are you ready to try and dance?" I start laughing.

"Seriously?" I ask.

"Of course Jenna! I'll run you through some steps," Margarita says.

She starts with some really simple body movements and steps. I watch her intently and try to follow along.

After a while we start some more complicated steps. "Jenna, look at yourself," my mom says. I take my eyes off Margarita and look at myself dancing in the mirror. It's the girl from the videos, it's the girl who was thriving, doing all the steps correctly and with elegance.

Wait, that's me. Right now. I am dancing. Not dancing at the bar (which I've been told I'm great at too) but actually following a simple routine and dancing.

A huge smile breaks out on my face and I start laughing. I wish I could bottle up this feeling that I have. I don't have memories of me dancing but I recognize this feeling. This is passion, this is me in my element. Dancing is my thing and I am so happy to be back doing it.

Margarita and I dance for a while, slowly building to even more complex steps. I'm able to follow it all and do it all. All of us are impressed. I just keep laughing with pure joy.

After a while, I get tired. I haven't moved like that since my stroke, but it feels so good.

"I think you should take lessons with me again. Let's do them this summer," Margarita says.

My eyes light up. “Are you serious? You would do that?” I ask.

“Yes! This is amazing. You already have your passion back just from that short time, I can tell. Let’s keep it going!” Margarita says.

I get the sense that this is what a kid feels like on Christmas morning. I just found my Christmas. Dancing is my Christmas.

Chapter 17

August 2022

My mom has taken a week off work. For the first half of the week, she got in her car and drove to wherever she felt like going. She texted me that she was safe but otherwise had no contact with the world. It was the breath of fresh air her soul needed after the past year.

She returned home halfway through the week and asked if I could flex my schedule a bit. The nature of my summer job allows me to work my hours when needed but also when I want to. I mostly interview and hire people for a September start. I had no interviews left for the week and just administrative stuff to do on my laptop, so I told my mom I could flex some time around other things.

She told me to pack a bag because we were going away for a few days.

And here we are in North Bay. My mom picked it as I have no idea where anything is besides Peterborough and now Toronto. My mom isn't sure why she chose North Bay, but here we are. We have spent the past two days lounging outside, me doing work and my mom reading. We work out in the hotel gym. We have gone for many walks to explore the area. We explored the Nipissing University campus, we hiked around a gorgeous waterfall (which nearly killed me but I did it!) and we ate good food together.

It has been relaxing and just what we both needed.

It is now our final night here in North Bay. I wrap up a meeting with my research team, and Mom and I decide to go to the beach for a bit before the sunset. We put on our bathing suits, grab our books, and head to the beach.

I lay my towel out on the sand. My mom starts to head to the water. "I'm going to swim," she says. The water hits her toes, and she recoils. "Oh, it's a bit colder than I thought," she laughs. "Jenna come on, swim with me," she says.

I really don't want to, I hate the cold, but how bad can it be? So I get up off my towel, take my shorts off and head towards the water.

My mom gets her phone and starts to video the moment, as she always does.

The water feels freezing cold. I decide I have to just run into the water quickly, like Julia and I did that day at the beach. Walking in slowly will be painful in the cold. I smile at my mom. "Here I go," I say.

I run into the water laughing at how cold it feels. When it gets to be around my waist, I dive into it, fully submersing myself.

But this feels different than any other water. I've lost which way is up. I feel like I'm spinning. Being pulled, crashing into things. *Wait, that must be the ground I'm crashing into. It's hard.* I try to feel it with my hand. My feet find it and I force my body up out of the water.

I wipe the water out of my eyes and peel my hair off my face as I frantically look around. Finally, behind me I see my mom standing there with her phone, still recording.

I must have only been under the water for a few seconds.

"What the fuck was that? The ocean just tried to kill me. I was just whipped around like a rag doll," I yell to my mom.

Her eyes grow wide. "Oh my gosh Jenna, I didn't even think about this. The undertow. The current. You've never swam in anything like that. You can't really swim. Fuck, I'm sorry hun. I forget sometimes this is all new to you," she says.

I stare back at her half laughing, half still freaking out. "Well, it's a good thing I figured it out. You would have just been standing there recording me drowning. 'Oh look how cute Jenna trying to swim is, everyone' meanwhile I'm dying and being thrown around," I say while laughing.

I walk out of the water and back to my mom. She hugs me and apologizes for forgetting about my lack of water knowledge and inability to swim well. We both laugh as she tries to shake the sand out of my knotted hair.

Eventually, my mom and I stop laughing. She says it's her turn to take a swim but she will actually swim and not drown. I go and sit on my towel and watch her glide through the water effortlessly. The current not attacking her as it did me. However, I do find the waves cool to watch. I think water is my happy place.

While sitting on my towel enjoying the warm sun, I begin to reflect a bit on what this learning experience has taught me. For one, I need to ramp up my swimming lessons. Bella and Ellen have been doing occasional swimming lessons with me in pools, and they have been going alright. My left side really struggles in the water, partly because the water is a new force working against it, and also because I can't see my left side to know how to move it in the water. I rely on watching my left arm and leg to make them move how I want until they get the motion. In water, it is hard to do this.

So maybe I need to look into more swimming lessons and ask Bella to take me to lakes and such where the water is not as controlled. My main goal is to not drown, and today that almost became a failed goal.

I reflect on how it is so funny that we all forget about my brain injury sometimes. My acquaintances often forget, as they haven't lived with me through this adventure. But my people are very on the ball at explaining new things or wanting to show something new to me. However, we all forget sometimes. Even I forget. The world truly does not stop for things like this. When my story went public during my hospital isolation, it was a quick reality of how the world works for me. For about two weeks I had thousands of messages every day, with people checking in, wanting updates, and just letting me know I had support. But then the next big thing came along and I was quickly forgotten about. Which I was okay with in a sense, as I'm not really one for being the main attraction.

However, this showed me that the world keeps going, and no one was going to accommodate me forever. No one was going to remember I suffered a stroke unless they saw me. No one would remember I had no memories unless I told them. So I realized that I needed to speak up for myself more, but also that we all forget.

Today, my mom not remembering I have never experienced an undertow before was not her fault, or mine. She didn't remember and I didn't know what it was to begin with. It's not anyone's fault and it worked out okay (minus some mild fear of the water now on my end - haha). But it just reminds me to ask questions more and to be more vocal about what I need. I don't want my stroke to become who I am, but I want to be able to ingest all the knowledge I can, and that takes explaining my situation and asking questions.

So I'm grateful when these forgetful moments do happen. They remind me of my situation and remind others, but also show me that we don't live in this constant state of focus on my stroke. I am still just Jenna to my people, and that feels great.

I enjoy the rest of the day in the sun, reading, laughing, eating, and researching swimming lessons in Peterborough.

* * *

My phone buzzes and I see it is a text from my friend Mark. He is here. I grab my backpack and yell to my mom upstairs "Mark is here."

I head outside to greet him. Mark and I are heading camping for the weekend! Jordan is coming up later tonight after work, but Mark and I are going to go and set up the campsite before dark. We say our goodbyes to my mom, load our food and such into the car and off we head.

Camping has been a huge part of my life. I grew up going camping every summer with my family but as Jordan and I got older we stopped going as much. Then when the pandemic hit, Jordan and I decided to start going camping again as something to do. So a core group of our friends started going yearly, with some other people coming sometimes and such.

Over the years it has turned into an annual thing for Jordan, Mark and me to go along with anyone else who wants to come.

Therefore with me not remembering camping, Jordan and Mark knew that we had to go again this year so I could re-learn what camping is.

So here we are.

Mark and I arrive at the campsite. We start by unloading everything out of his car. Mark goes to the front camp store to grab ice while I start laying everything out. I find the tent and unpack it, confused but ready to put it up. Mark comes back and we dump ice into the coolers.

Then we tackle the tent set-up together. "This is actually way easier than I thought. Jordan will be so impressed with us," Mark laughs. The tent turns out to be easily set up as the poles are already assembled and it just requires a few button clicks to pop it right up. Jordan had expressed their doubt about our abilities in a loving way, but Mark and I do exceptionally well.

"Well, might as well get the camping spirit going to give you the full experience now that set-up is complete," Mark said as he throws me a beer.

And that is how the rest of the weekend went.

We drank, we swam, played spikeball and football, had fires in the evening with card games and laughs. We even had some of our friends from our baseball team join us, and Logan and Pat came to visit. It was a great weekend and I did in fact learn I love camping still.

When we returned from our camping adventures, August was almost over, which meant it was very shortly time for my birthday. On the actual day of my birthday, I kept things very chill as it stressed me out a bit. I let myself sleep in, worked from home, and just relaxed. Later in the day, Pat brought me French fries (one of my favourite foods) to celebrate our day together as we share the same birthday. Then Julia came home from work and brought me a cupcake. After enjoying my cupcake, we headed to dinner with my mom before our dance lessons. It was a perfect day.

However, besides just my actual birthday, on the following weekend Jordan made me have a party. This time being my actual birthday and not my half-birthday from February, I was having more of an adult party. Friends came to my house and we hung out on my back porch. Aunt Sandi even baked me a drunken unicorn cake for the occasion! Later in the evening we headed to a bar and enjoyed the night dancing and playing pool.

Overall August was a busy month with lots of new firsts that I loved. However, a lot of those included moments that are special to me and my people, which I am choosing to keep between us (also because of the alcohol involved in some - haha). But I think these general ideas are important to share with you all as I am appreciative for celebrating another year of my life.

Chapter 18

September 2022

"Hey Jen, look! The leaves are starting to change," my mom says.

"Huh?" I look at her, confused. I glance out the car window at the trees. They look like the same old trees I've seen for months.

My mom looks back at me. "You know. The leaves. They are changing colours. Fall? Hello?" she says. I stare back at her, completely lost.

"Oh shit! Fall! Jenna you don't know what fall is!" she says. "You remember Kara going over the seasons with you in speech therapy? Remember how after summer comes fall. Well, the leaves change colour and fall off the trees, so they are bare for the winter. It gets really beautiful! They turn red and orange and yellow, and it all looks gorgeous," my mom explains to me.

I turn and look closer at the trees. Maybe there are a few leaves that are different. I don't get it but I add it to my daily list of things I don't know but will look up before bed.

Fall. Interesting.

"I'm sorry I forget sometimes," my mom apologizes.

"It's okay. I forget too and, truthfully, I don't even know these things exist unless you tell me, so I'm not upset, just confused about this world I live in," I say with a slight smile. We ride the rest of the way in quiet, me thinking about this new idea that fall isn't just a label for a few months; it actually means something.

* * *

A couple days later I am still thinking about fall.

My supervisor, lab-mates and I are unpacking some computer equipment. We unpack all the boxes and set up the new computer lab.

"Do a few of you mind helping me carry these boxes out to the recycling?" my supervisor asks.

"Sure," I say while grabbing some of the boxes.

My lab-mate, supervisor and I take the boxes outside to the recycling. We start walking back towards the building.

"Look, that tree's leaves are starting to change," my lab-mate says.

"Ugh, that means summer is ending," my supervisor says.

"Do you not like fall?" My lab-mate asks him.

"I don't dislike it, it just means summer is over and winter is coming," he explains.

"Fair enough, Jenna do you like fall?" my lab-mate asks.

"Um, I'm not sure. I don't know. I'm just excited to experience it for the first time," I say.

Both my supervisor and lab-mate stop walking and stare at me. "What do you mean you don't know what fall is? You've lived here before. You were here last year in the fall," my supervisor says.

"Yeah, but I can't remember it. My stroke happened in December. I don't remember fall," I explain.

"Wait. You can't even remember fall?" my supervisor asks.

"No. Like I'm telling you, I don't remember anything before December," I say.

"Shit. I'm sorry, I didn't realize you didn't remember that much. That's like your whole episodic memory wiped. Semantic. Woah. I didn't know. I need to look into this," my supervisor exclaims. In this moment his understanding of where I am at, brilliant, but missing a lot of background knowledge, became a blessing for the future.

This, however, became a personal pivotal moment as well. I always knew people do not and won't understand when I say I can't remember anything. They think 'oh okay, you don't remember who I am or your childhood.' But no. It's so much more than that. Not knowing what fall is, or that it even is a thing, is my reality. This is a perfect example to get people to at least try to understand what the world is like for me. I often think to myself that I wish I could put people into my brain for an hour. To have them understand how I see the world because I don't know how or have the words to explain it. Fall is probably the closest I will get to people's understanding.

* * *

"Before we start into multiple regression, I thought we could take a minute and say what our favourite thing is about fall," my professor says to the class.

Instantly I start sweating. I already feel dumb compared to everyone in this class. How am I going to admit that I don't know what fall is? The panic is unreal.

My classmates start throwing out their favourite things, the leaf colours, the fall smell, fall foods such as soup and chili. I'm overly confused. The smell of fall? Chili? What are these things? Everyone says something. I keep my eyes glued to the table, sweating and fighting back tears.

My professor doesn't directly ask me, which I am so thankful for. But it feels obvious I didn't contribute. There are only 12 of us in this univariate statistics class. And I'm the dumb girl that doesn't know what any of the statistics we talk about are, let alone what my favourite thing about fall is.

My mind is spinning with how these people think I'm dumb, how they find me a loser, and how they only talk to me out of pity. How everyone else knows so much. How I don't deserve to be here. What am I even doing with my life?

I stand up and quickly walk out of the class. I dart down the hallway to the bathroom. I lock myself in a stall and the tears pour down my face. I can't breathe.

I feel like I want to scream at myself for being so dumb, but also I just want to disappear under water. I have never felt anxiety and shame like this. I am struggling so hard with the transition back to school. I feel like the odd one out in my cohort. It's a small group of us and everyone is so nice. But I have been so in my head about it all. I am judging myself; I'm ashamed of myself and my brain injury. I feel like I don't deserve this life. I feel as if everyone else is so much better and more prepared than me. I feel inadequate and useless. I still don't know my alphabet in order, I am failing this statistic course, I am struggling to make friends openly. I really thought I would excel in my Master's, like it was meant to be. But it has become a huge source of anxiety in my life. I dread going to school. On Sunday nights I find myself unable to sleep, puking with worry. In class I find myself fighting tears, running to the bathroom to cry.

This isn't me. Who have I become?

* * *

"Hi, Jenna. It's so nice to meet you," Amanda says.

"It's nice to meet you too. Thank you for seeing me," I reply.

"No problem at all. I'm glad you're here. I think for today we will chat for a bit and then I'll give you a tour of the place and show you our neuro rooms so you know what it will look like next time you come in. Does that sound alright?" she asks.

"Yeah. That sounds great," I reply.

"Great. So let's start with a little bit about you and your story. I know we've talked a bit, but do you mind running me through everything again?" Amanda asks.

I launch into the story of my stroke, my rehab journey, and my still-present struggles. I discuss how I am severely struggling with school, and feeling unworthy. Struggling with being present in my life, and how I'm scared of these feelings. I explain that is what has led me to be here today, led me to seek therapy.

Amanda and I go through a bunch of questions and talk about some of my current issues. We discuss what I want out of this process. And we decide that I will do a combination of talk therapy along with neurofeedback training.

I agree to try neurofeedback for my cognition. I have no idea if it will work, or if it will have any effect on my energy, concentration and attention, or even my memory. But I figure anything is worth a try at this point.

A few nights ago, I went home from school and completely broke down with my roommate, Heather. We had a really serious conversation about me moving forward and getting okay with myself and with school again. I used to love school, and I wanted to get back to that. Heather and I agreed that maybe it was time I reached out to a therapist. I found a local place that had experience with brain injuries, and they also did neurofeedback. I did some research and even with mixed reviews I figured I might as well try neurofeedback. It had been months since I did any professional rehab work so maybe it was time I tried a new avenue to see if there is progression. So I reached out, and my therapy journey began again.

I also have been trying to become more myself at school. Instead of just hiding out and working in my lab where I feel safe, I am trying to connect with other students more. Pat and I went out for drinks with a gal from my cohort and her partner. We had a great time, and I was pleasantly surprised that she seemed to like me so much. I really thought everyone thought I was the stupid girl. But it turns out I was wrong.

I have been really private about my stroke with the students in my cohort because I don't want them to think differently about me. However, at drinks, I had the opportunity to share my story, and it went well. I was asked where I grew up and what it was like. I had looked to Pat with panic as I struggled to answer, "Guelph" and not "Guelph Goddamit" as I always say. Pat gave me a small smile and asked, "Do you guys know about Jenna's story?"

I started freaking out. Everyone had always been nice and receptive to my story, but I had it in my head that my classmates would judge me for it.

When they said they didn't know it and looked to me, Pat gave me a reassuring smile, and I started to give the short story. Pat jumped in and started explaining how far I had come from a few months ago. Their faces dropped.

"Wait. You are telling me that less than a year ago you had a stroke and here you are doing your Master's?" my classmate asked me.

"Yeah, I guess," I said shyly.

"Holy shit. You are amazing! I can't believe that," she replied.

I felt my body physically relax. I didn't even realize how tense I was. I smiled a little and said thanks.

Pat looked at me and said, "See, it's okay. You are amazing hun."

From that moment on it began to feel like I had an ally at school. My classmate started to take time to explain things to me, to make sure I always understood what people were saying, to explain stats to me. She became a really good friend.

The walls I had built inside my mind lost a few bricks of resistance. Maybe these people weren't all judging me that hard, maybe they didn't hate or pity me. Maybe it would be okay, because I had a friend.

Chapter 19

October 2022

"It's so nice to meet you!" I say when I log onto the meeting. Lisa agrees that it's nice to meet me as well.

"It was so nice to hear from you. I'm so excited about the potential of this project. Why don't you start with telling me a bit about your story?" Lisa says.

I jump into my usual speech about who I am and what has happened to me. I talk about my rehab journey and how far I've come, and how much further I want to go. When I finish, I pause and take a second to look at Lisa's reaction.

I notice tears in her eyes.

"Wow. I'm blown away. This story is amazing; it needs to be told. If you are willing to work with me, then we will get your story out there," Lisa says to me.

A huge smile breaks out onto my face. I have a publisher. Someone wants to publish my story, my book. This crazy project I've started is becoming a reality.

I'm blown away and overwhelmed with gratefulness.

My story is going to be told, I just need to finish creating it.

* * *

I am finding holidays to be hard. They are overwhelming, stressful, and given too high a degree of expectations.

Thanksgiving is new to me. My family typically celebrates Freedom Day on Thanksgiving weekend, as we celebrate who we have become and the strength we have had since my dad left us. I've learned that in the past we have always gone for a trail hike on this weekend, we spend time together, and one year we even got tattoos of strength to celebrate 5 years. However, besides a nice walk together, this year is a little different as Jordan is away with some previously made plans. Therefore, this year my mom and I had a Thanksgiving gathering with Ron and Ellen, and Ellen's extended family.

On Thanksgiving I liked the food, I enjoyed the time off school and work, but it was stressful just the same. I don't understand the holidays and why they happen. I've been told the backstory of them numerous times, yet they still confuse me.

I find the gatherings on holidays hard. They are loud and a lot on my head. Thanksgiving was hard for this but I coped as best as I could, given what I was dealt.

It's Halloween today.

I went to my lab dressed up as my supervisor. It was fun to dress up like that, and he thought it was a hilarious surprise. This holiday seems a little less stressful than others.

I just got to Bella's with Heather. I had gone home from the lab and changed out of my costume, and was now beginning my friend's Halloween events.

Bella, Heather, Julia, and I all are at Bella's place for the festivities.

"Alright, go throw your costume on and let's do this!" Bella says.

Julia and I go change. Once we are ready Heather hands us each a pillowcase and sends us out the door.

Bella and Julia start walking down the driveway with me. We cross the street to the neighbour's house.

"What do we do when we get there?" I ask.

"Well, there is either going to be a bowl of candy on the porch and you can take a piece of candy, or you have to knock on the door and say trick or treat when the person answers so they give you candy," Julia explains.

"And the golden rule is if the lights are on in the house you can go but if the house is dark then they aren't participating," Bella adds.

"So we just go to all these houses and take candy from random people?" I ask while laughing.

"Yeah basically," Julia and Bella laugh.

We get to the neighbour's front door. I see a bowl of candy sitting on the porch. I look at Bella and Julia. They nod and grab a piece to show me how to do it.

I grab a piece of candy and put it into my pillowcase bag.

"Yeah! Just like that dude," Bella says.

I smile. "Okay and now we just go to the next?" I ask.

"Yup. We just keep going to houses until we are tired or it's too late," Julia says.

"This is so weird but okay," I say, laughing with the girls.

We walk to the next house. We get to the porch but I don't see a bowl of candy. I look to the girls feeling nervous about what to do.

"Want me to do this one?" Julia asks.

"Yes please, I'm nervous."

"Okay, but make your voice higher when you talk - haha. Remember we have to be little kids," Bella reminds me.

Julia knocks on the door. After a minute a lady opens the door and says "Happy Halloween!"

"Trick or treat," Julia and Bella say. I smile at this moment; next time I'll say it with them.

We go to many houses and repeat these same actions. After a while, it starts to rain so we head back to Bella's house.

When we get there Heather is waiting for us. We dump all our candy out on the floor, and the girls show me how to sort it like we would as kids. They also start trading candy with each other, and offering me trades. I'm starting to get a headache from this excitement but take a moment to just sit quietly and enjoy the moment.

"Alright dude I can tell you're getting tired. We have one more place we have to go tonight, so let's do it now before you crash," Bella says.

We put our shoes back on and head out to the car. Heather heads home as she has a headache, but Julia and I climb into Bella's car. We drive a few short minutes to our next neighbourhood. We go trick or treating at a few houses. We are laughing and joking loudly. As we approach the house, Pat steps out from the neighbour's driveway.

"Do I know those voices?" he asks.

"Trick or treat!" we all say while laughing.

"This is amazing! Look at you guys!" Pat exclaims while laughing. "Here, come with me, I got stuff for you."

We head with Pat up to his front porch. He brings us a few bowls of candy and we pick through, taking a fair share. He also offers us a beer, which is quite rewarding after this night.

Pat lets his dog, Bauer, outside for us to see. We play with Bauer and eat candy while laughing on his front porch. We show him our onesie costumes that we threw together earlier tonight. Bella is a dinosaur, Julia is a fox, and I am a moose.

After a while, we get all get cold and tired. We say our goodbyes to Pat and Bauer, and head back to Bella's car. When we make it back to Bella's place we change into dry, warm clothes and finish trading our candy.

My head is really hurting at this point and I'm exhausted. Julia suggests we head home so we pack up our candy. When we get home, I show Heather my candy with excitement. We find a bowl to put my candy in.

My trick-or-treat excitement has started to wear off and the headache gets more intense. I quickly get ready for bed and fall fast asleep, pleasantly surprised at how well this holiday went.

Chapter 20

November 2022

Julia is knocking on my door. "Jenna, are you awake?" she says.

I roll over and say, "Yeah, I'm awake, just don't want to get up. You can open my door."

It's 6:00 am and Julia just got home from work as I am getting up to head into lab.

Julia comes into my room. "Jenna, it snowed! Get up, put clothes on, we are going outside," she says.

I sit up quickly and look out my window. I see the white. Fresh snow! The first snowfall.

"Snow!" I yell, and then quiet down with a laugh as the rest of my roommates are still asleep.

I jump out of bed, quickly get dressed and run downstairs to meet Julia.

We both get our boots and coats on quickly. Julia hands me a pair of gloves. “Put these on, it will be cold,” she instructs me.

We head outside. I step onto our porch and take in the scene in front of me. I feel overwhelmed with the view.

I don’t remember the first snowfall last year as it probably happened before my stroke. My first memory of snow is when we got a bad storm and no one could get to see me last January. I had laid flat on my hospital bed and watched the snow fall from the sky in the little opening at the top of my window. I stared at it for hours that night, imagining what it must have felt like and looked like in the winter wonderland outside the boarded window. When I woke up that next morning, there was a small amount of snow that had collected between the windows and the boards. It was like the world was gifting me with a little view of what the rest of the world looked like.

This morning, Julia grabs my left arm and I grab the railing with my right hand.

“It’s going to be slippery. You have to be careful,” Julia says as we walk down our front steps.

I get onto the front lawn and shuffle my feet, feeling the slippery snow beneath me.

“Here, feel it,” Julia says as she bends down and scoops up a handful of snow.

I take my glove off and she dumps it into my hand. It's cold and wet. "Throw it up, it's fun," Julia says.

I throw it up and it floats down onto us. We both start laughing. Tears spring into my eyes as I notice snow starting to fall from the sky all around us. I'm overwhelmed with emotions. It's beautiful and I'm alive to experience it.

Julia gives me a quick 5-minute rundown on how to drive in the snow, and how to take it slow. She explains how it can take longer to break so I need to go slower and give myself more time to slow down. "You know how it's slippery for you to walk in; well, it's slippery like that for your car too, even with your snow tires. So just take it slow and give lots of space to break and for other drivers, as sometimes it's more them you have to watch out for," Julia says with a wink.

Then she shows me how to brush snow off my car. I already learned how to scrape it off by watching how-to videos in my driveway one morning at 7 am before trying to get to school. But now Julia shows me how to brush the snow off without getting it all over myself. It's different than scraping the frost and I'm grateful for her lesson.

"Tonight I'll show you how to shovel as well!" Julia says with a laugh.

When my driving lesson wraps up we practice shuffling in the snow so I can walk by myself without her help. It's different for me to walk in boots, let alone boots and slippery ground.

After I practice walking for a few minutes Julia and I take another moment to just enjoy the weather.

We laugh, we throw the snow at each other, and we jump around arm-in-arm under the falling flakes.

I'm sure if any neighbours are looking outside we appear crazy, as we laugh and cry in the snow at 6 am on a Wednesday morning, but we don't care. For us, this is pure joy.

* * *

I often hear people say things such as it takes a village. It takes a village to raise a child, it takes a village to get through tough things. But truly it's amazing to feel that village form around you. I started recognizing I was having serious trouble in my univariate statistics class a couple of weeks ago when my marks reflected I was failing. I knew I was struggling before but now with getting actual marks back, the reality is setting in of how poorly it is going. I brought it up to my supervisor and immediately my village started to take form. My supervisor and I formed a plan of attack for the semester. We put my thesis research on hold until after my stats class finished. We changed our weekly thesis meetings to weekly stats lectures. Our lab meetings began to have a component of stats knowledge taught in them as well. My supervisor has become a huge part of my village.

In a seminar with other grad students, I started talking to a second-year Master's student who I knew from the previous school year. He was aware of my situation. I expressed my trouble with stats and he jumped into my village. He took me to a Ph.D. student and connected the two of us. The Ph.D. student agreed to mentor me in software coding. The students in my program quickly became my village.

It is not unusual for me to enter my house after school with tears drying on my face from my drive home. The girls are used to me being overwhelmed from the day and just purely drained, resulting in a loss of emotional control. However, they are always quick to jump in and ask me about my day and to point me toward the positives. One day in our normal routine, I spilled to Julia about my rough time with stats. Julia immediately stepped in and grew into another component of my village. She went to her room, pulled out all her undergraduate course notes, went with me to my room and found mine and said, "Let's learn stats again bud."

Between two sets of old notes, two textbooks, seven rivers of tears, three bottles of Advil for my headaches, some occasional wine, and three 'tutors,' my village and I almost got me through my statistics courses.

In my coding course, I am doing quite well; however, the univariate statistics course is not so great still.

"I don't mean to be rude, but I think you need to hear this. You are failing the course. Anything below 80% in grad school is considered a fail. You are failing and this could seriously harm your chances of getting into a Ph.D. program. I think the problem is that you are doing so well given your circumstances that it feels like you're so close, but you are failing the course Jenna," my supervisor says.

And sadly it is true, and I do need to hear this.

"Yeah, I know you're right and I needed to hear this. Thank you. I think I should drop the course and we figure out alternative options, either taking it next year or a different course or something," I reply.

"That is probably the best. Next year think of how much further you will be in re-learning stats and then you can not only pass the course but excel in it. I think you're making the right choice. It's hard but I'm proud of how hard you tried. You really are exceptional," my supervisor praises.

We wrap up our meeting and I send the emails I need to send to start the process of dropping the course. It's a tough decision but I remind myself I'm not a failure, I'm just planning for my future. I am doing amazing in my other course, so I will be able to excel in this one too, once I'm ready to take it, once I learn more of the background knowledge again.

Sometimes these moments humble me. I struggle deeply with failure and a fear of failure. My sibling Jordan and I have talked about how my father always expected me to fail, and told me that I would. To him, I was the pretty one, the one who would flirt my way through life. I would excel because I had the looks to do it. But this is not me. I am intelligent, I am driven beyond what one could imagine, and I am successful because I work my ass off. Even though I don't have these memories of my father, I have dreams about it and I still carry the emotions and the scars.

So for me to drop this course feels like giving in to failure. To admit I can't do it, that I can't get an 80% when my average sits in the 90s, is crushing.

My supervisor knows this, which is why he gave me the truth bluntly, as I was opposed to telling it to myself. But he also has been and will be there every single step of the way through this.

So at this moment, I remind myself that sometimes we need to fail at things. Sometimes it's good for us. It can remind us about what we have accomplished and what we have yet to accomplish.

Univariate statistics is a hard course for most. And here I am; less than a year ago I was paralyzed, incapable of talking, incapable of knowing my own name, of knowing anything around me, and I almost completed this course.

I start to feel a little piece of respect for myself that I've been working hard to find.

Respect for who I am, and what I have done.

* * *

Admitting I am failing statistics has not been the only hard time during this semester of school.

When I started to become more mobile in the hospital, my mom and I would tour around the hallways, as it's quite boring being in a hospital for two months. As I started to become more cognitively aware of my surroundings and of social norms, I noticed something weird. Anytime my mom and I would go to the main floor of the hospital and grab a coffee or such, people would stare. It was like I was a freak and they were observing me.

There were times when I understood why people were staring at me. I would have moments in the first few months where I couldn't control my filter and would get what I call 'stroke brain.' I would be yelling at people that they were 'fucking dingos' or clicking my tongue really loudly over and over.

Or even as Jordan loves to recall, I kept screaming 'chuck snow at your head' one time while getting a coffee after learning about snow and what to do with it.

So yes, in these situations I would probably stare at me as well.

But now, where I am at with my recovery, I'm not used to the awkward behaviour of others.

For example, I don't use my wheelchair as much anymore. Partly because I'm able to function without it and partly because I avoid using it when I should, as it's awkward and embarrassing.

I struggle to grocery shop still and should use my wheelchair to do it. But when I do, it's always uncomfortable. I've had people interject as my friends and I are in mid-conversation about what apples to get. They ask my friends, "What's wrong with her?" even though I'm sitting right there. I've had people crash their carts into displays because they are staring at me and not paying attention to where they are going.

I've had people run across the room during a lecture, making everyone turn and stare, so they can open the door for me to leave when my friend was about to quietly open it for me. I've even had random people (especially older men) make comments such as, "Eh no running for you then - haha."

Even recently I went to Toronto for an event with some friends. I used my wheelchair as it was busy and we had a lot of standing time. My friend Emma turned to me and said, "Is this actually what it is like for you? Cause holy shit people are weird. Staring, walking into things, avoiding you like the plague. I'm so sorry you deal with this. I'm so uncomfortable."

Pat always tells me people stare because I'm such a pretty lady. Which makes me laugh and takes away a bit of the uncomfortable feelings.

I get that people stare at things that are different, but I just didn't think a wheelchair was that out of the ordinary.

These events deter me from using the supports I need, and from admitting I need help. I'm not confident with my disability.

Therefore, when I received an email informing me that in my research seminar for school, our research pitch presentations are being moved outside the classroom to a nature hike format, I felt panicked.

The concept is that we will hike the Drumlin trail on Trent's campus and stop at a few designated stations for first-year students to present our 60-second research pitches.

My panic is not about the pitch. I have been preparing for weeks and I actually quite enjoy public speaking. I even know I'm not half bad at it from when I gave the conference presentation in June. The real issue is the hike.

Upon receiving the email, I immediately go to my village of people. I ask the girls if any of them are free on Friday. Bella is.

I email my professor and ask if it would be alright if my friend came for the hike to help me do it. He responds by saying yes, and also that I don't have to do the hike if I don't want to.

But it's me. Of course I'm going to try. Plus I don't want to be the only one that doesn't pitch that day as I've already dropped the statistics course that the rest of the first years are in. I already feel a bit of an outcast. I can't not do this mandatory pitch as well.

I email back saying that I will try the hike, I request that I be put earlier on the list of presenters so I can back out if needed, and that my friend and I will get through it together.

On the morning of the hike, I become quite anxious. My supervisor and I alter my pitch a little, which is stressful. But mostly I am nervous as it is raining and everything is going to be wet and slippery for this hike.

My supervisor comes into the lab and asks me why I am so agitated. He explains that I seem really off, so I tell him about my hiking concerns. His eyes grow wide as he says, “Oh shit, I didn’t even think about you doing the hike and having any problems. You walk so well in here, I didn’t even think it would be an issue. But not even with you in mind, I told the professors that they can’t do the hike. It’s inaccessible to begin with for everyone. So stop stressing, you guys are just going to walk on the grass trail around the drumlin; it’s flat and just grass.”

I explain to him how I appear to walk fine because I don’t walk long distances at the lab and it’s all flat and even flooring. People notice my walking struggles when the ground is uneven or slippery, and when I walk for a long time and get tired.

The afternoon rolls around, and Bella picks me up from my lab and drives me to the other side of campus. I explain how apparently the hike is off but I am still happy she is there to support me.

We get to the meeting spot outside the drumlin and I feel awkward. I love having Bella with me, but I can tell everyone is confused about who this is and why she is here.

I remind myself that it's okay that I need help, and that I'm so grateful Bella is willing to do this.

We wait a few minutes for all the professors and grad students to show up. Only the first years have to pitch their research, but it is mandatory for all the psychology grad students to show up. Even some undergraduates have come to observe.

When everyone is there, the professor running the hike announces that they did the hike this morning and it isn't too wet so we will be hiking the trail.

I look at Bella with sheer panic. She reassures me that we are going to get through it.

The group starts walking, and Bella and I take to the end, knowing we will be slower.

The first little bit is alright as the ground is flat, but then we start to go up the hill on the trail. Down the middle, the trail is sheer ice. On the sides the trail is mud. Bella tells me to go on the mud, and she walks half on the ice, half in the mud beside me. She stands on my left side and we link arms. I'm death gripping her as she supports half my weight.

"I'm so sorry. I'm really struggling to walk," I say to Bella.

"Dude this is nothing. I would push your wheelchair up this if I had to. Let's do it," Bella replies.

As we trail along, one of the professors yells down to me asking if I'm okay, with a look of concern. I look up at them and see everyone staring down at me as Bella and I hobble up the hill. I'm mortified and imagining everything they all are thinking but I force myself to say, 'I'm good" back to the professor and I put my head back down.

We watch a few people fall on the ice and I pray that we don't go down.

Finally, we reach the first stop and the first two people give their pitches. They get hooked up to the media person's microphone, introduce themselves and do their pitch. Questions are asked and then we continue the hike.

I tell myself it wasn't a big deal and that I can so do this.

Bella and I are almost at the second station where everyone is waiting for us. It's my turn to pitch. We finally get there and I feel exhausted but ready.

The two professors in charge come up to me as I arrive.

"You don't have to do this. You can just go," they say.

I look at them confused and look to Bella who is equally as confused.

"If it's too hard, just go. You don't have to pitch," they say.

"But if I don't pitch, I don't pass the course? What do you mean I'm not pitching?" I ask.

"No it's fine, you don't have to. Just go back. You don't have to do this. We can even just have a conversation here about your research loudly but not a formal pitch to everyone. Just tell me about your research right now and that's good enough. You don't need everyone to hear," they say.

I look around and everyone is staring at us. Tears start to well up in my eyes. "I'm pitching," I say as I grab Bella's arm and walk past them to the middle of the crowd to pitch.

I feel confused, embarrassed, and overwhelmed.

The professors follow me as they see I've made up my mind. One of them stands beside me. They tell the media guy to not record anything, adding to my confusion. Then they gesture to me and start to introduce me to the group, who already knows me.

"This is Jenna, a first-year Master's student with some amazing research you all should hear about. Jenna has some really exceptional circumstances but is still with us here today so we should all be so proud."

I'm fighting back the tears. I am so embarrassed. No one else got an introduction, no one else has the right to announce my circumstances. I don't want everyone to think differently of me or treat me differently. But they all must think I'm crazy right now.

I look at Bella, she looks super angry but also empathetic for me. We make eye contact and she gives me a small nod as if to say 'you can do it, I'm here.'

So I look to the crowd and I start to pitch my research.

After the first couple of lines, the one professor says, "Ahh good point," and I lose my thought.

My mind goes blank and I can't think of the next line. All my words leave.

I start to cry. I point to my head and keep repeating "Stuck, stuck. It stuck." Not even able to form actual sentences.

I'm crying, my aphasia and stutter in full force. I don't want to exist at this moment.

The professor who interrupted me asks me a question to try and help. It all comes back. I thank him and finish my pitch.

When I finish my friends in the program who know my situation cheer as loud as they can, chanting my name. I appreciate the encouragement but truthfully I have never wanted not to be seen more in my life. I have never felt this level of shame and vulnerability. It reminds me of the first time a nurse showered me. Absolute vulnerability and shame.

Eventually, we move on and finish the hike. The professors told me I did amazing and that my supervisor would be proud. I want to puke.

I am not the least bit proud of myself, and am so grateful that my supervisor was not there to witness that. I appreciate the professors trying to help me. I personally believe that they realized how big of a mistake they made with the hike once they saw me trying to do it. It's amazing to me the difference between when people see me normally and when they see my disability. I'm not mad at the professors, I'm just embarrassed. My classmates must think I'm crazy, that I have severe social anxiety or fear of presenting. It is okay if I did, but I'm embarrassed because I actually love presenting and do well with it. So for this to happen as it has is a major letdown. And again my disability made me a freak to everyone else. It's the same feelings as when I use my wheelchair again after not using it for a while and I forget the stares and comments. It's the same feelings as when people laugh at me because I don't know what something common is and I don't want to explain my circumstances. It's the same feelings I often have out in this world that I struggle to belong in.

I'm not mad people act this way with me, I don't even judge them for it or hold it against them. It's just the way the world works. I just wish my life was different sometimes, easier, not as vulnerable. I just wish I fit more into this world that I feel like I know nothing about.

After the hike, all my classmates go out for a drink together. I decline the offer. I go home and cry.

Chapter 21

December 11, 2022

My stroke-iversary.

1 year.

12 months.

365 days.

A year ago I began the journey of a lifetime.

I was partially paralyzed, acquired severe retrograde amnesia, lost my ability to talk, and developed a stutter and aphasia.

Intense rehab, speech therapy and cognition work. Learning to say 'Hi Mom,' learning to stand, to use a wheelchair, wiggle my fingers, pick up a fork, shower myself, walk, climb stairs, live independently again and so much more.

Discovering who Jenna Dakin is. What I am. What I like, what I don't like. Who I was before, who I am now. Learning what has changed about me since my stroke. Learning that I don't need to find myself in this world, but rather create myself.

Exploring this world I woke up in but don't belong to. Learning who my people are, and what other humans even are. Finding out norms and cultures. Histories and futures. Repairing 21 years of lost memories.

365 days of learning with years of knowledge still to come.

Today has been hard. My celebratory plans got cancelled due to the weather, people forgot about my day, and I was more emotional than I expected.

It wasn't spent how I wanted but it made me reflect.

There is no perfect way to celebrate this. A year ago everyone, including myself, thought I was going to die. Thought my brain was shutting down. That I was losing all neurological function. But I didn't. I am here and I am excelling. What is the perfect way to celebrate that?

It's 11 days into this month and it's already been great.

I got to go to a concert. Emma, Jordan, Andrew and I went to see The Trews play. I absolutely love them. I've had a deep connection with music as soon as Jordan showed me what Spotify was way back in January.

Music stayed in my brain through my stroke. I remember it. And in a sense, it feels like one of my closest friends. It's a reminder that the Jenna I was before is still kinda here, waiting for me to discover. It's emotional and it gives me an outlet for my emotions. Sometimes I can't name what I'm feeling. I can't explain to people what it's like to be me in this world, but when I play certain songs, I can feel my emotions in them and know that maybe I'm not so alone.

The Trews, The Glorious Sons, Zac Brown Band, John Legend, P!nk, Tom Odell, Hozier, Tones and I, 5SOS, The Struts, Lady Gaga, The Lumineers, Rage Against The Machine, and even Snoop Dogg singing the alphabet all made my top 2022 songs. I love it, everything I listen to I love.

Seeing The Trews was probably one of the best times I've had this year. I sang every word, and everyone else in the room disappeared, it was just me and the music.

I now know that every concert I can go to, I will. Music is my outlet.

And so has been this book.

I started this book out of anger, out of hurt. A lot of people told me I should write a book because I'm an inspiration. I think that's a load of bull. I see myself as a girl with goals who will do what it takes to achieve them.

But I lost a friend along the way this past year. A friend was upset by something I did and they went to someone else about it. This other person told me what I had done wrong, treated me like I was quite stupid because of my brain injury, and also informed me that because of my stroke, my friend had no idea how to talk to me about it as they didn't know how I would react. I messaged my friend saying I'm still me and I value our friendship enough that they can talk to me about issues. I never got a response.

This really caught me off guard. These two people who I love, and who I thought had my back, really isolated me and treated me like a brain injury rather than just me, whether they meant to or not.

So in my hurt, I sat down that night quite emotional and said 'Fuck it.' And I wrote. I wrote, and wrote, and wrote, and then it was 2 am. And I realized my tears had dried and I felt okay.

And it hit me. Writing is therapeutic to me. When I was isolated in the hospital and I wrote my feelings and my anger out, I felt so much better. I don't always have the words to speak but I have the words to write.

And the next thing I knew I was halfway through writing a book and starting to consider publishing it. My goal as I wrote became therapy. But as I started to consider publication, some other goals formed. What if this book can bring someone into my mind, and show what it's like for me in this world? What if someone else out there knows what this is like? What if I can help someone who can't write to be able to know they aren't alone? What if I can get help? What if a doctor or researcher reads this and can help me or at least attempt to? What if I can study myself more? All the what-ifs started to form and it became more of a drive to finish the book. So I kept writing.

When beginning writing I thought starting the book was hard. Once my goals formed it seemed that writing it was easy. But as I got closer to the end, I realized that finishing it is harder. I have a huge list of things I wanted to write about but didn't fit in. It's been hard to decide what to include. What is interesting to read, what is boring, what is too personal, and what do people actually care about? My publisher, Lisa, and I came up with an outline for my book. When I made the outline it came out to 21 chapters. I didn't plan for this but it felt right. My stroke happened at 21, in 2021. It was a meaningful coincidence so I knew I had to keep it to 21 chapters as I finished writing.

I wish I could drone on forever about all the things I've learned this year, but truthfully I could write this for the rest of my life then. I wanted to include things such as learning about boats when Pat took me boating this summer, my Aunt Sandi showing me how to bake cupcakes, my Uncle Ken giving me car mechanic lessons, doing swimming lessons, more about my dance lessons, making friends at baseball, falling in love with teaching at school even with my aphasia moments, ruining Easter by getting Covid, or even going with Jordan to Nova Scotia when they moved there. But there just isn't enough room for it all.

I had the idea of writing a list of all these inspirational things I've learned this past year to wrap up this book. But after writing my second one down, I realized there isn't this great list of inspirational things I can pull out. My life is ordinary to me. It's not inspirational, it's just my life. I wake up every morning, go about my routine and learn some stuff along the way. So yes, I could write my list about how not to be a dick to disabled people or how I manage to balance two degrees while writing a book, or how I am so grateful I get to experience all these firsts again, but truthfully I'm not going to change the world with this. I'm not inspirational in my telling with a list; my story is what will help people. My story is what I came here to write, and that is what I did. I focused on my learning of the world, learning who I am, and learning who I want to be.

Truthfully, I will never stop learning, just as everyone else doesn't stop learning. My learning might be a little different but it's the same journey everyone else is taking, just a different timeline.

The piece about this book that I love is that it is a little bit of insight into my brain. I have expressed throughout this book and in my daily life that I wish people could go inside my head for an hour and understand what it is like. This book is probably as close as I am going to get. It gives you a small glimpse into what my life has been like, and it's a reminder for me. My medical team has no idea what is wrong with me, or what caused this. Could it happen again? Absolutely. Could I lose my memories again? Absolutely.

But I will always have this book. This piece of therapy. This look into the first year of my new life.

I will never be the same person I was. Things have changed in terms of my personality, and my likes and dislikes, and I have a completely new experience to live with. I will never be fully recovered in my opinion, as I just don't see that as possible with where I am at. I'm damn proud of where I am at, but I also know there will always be things that are different for me.

However, this past year, this past 21 chapters of my life have been the absolute best first year of my life that I could have imagined. I've learned so much, I've done so much, I've felt every emotion I think possible, and I've started to become who I want to be. I've started to create myself and be the Jenna I aspire to be.

21 Cups has been therapeutic. A reflectionary piece, a guilt-releasing, strength-building and eye-opening experience. I chose 21 Cups as the title as 21 seemed so fitting. And anyone who was around last year when this happened knows that truly everything was called a cup to me. Cups were my life for a while.

21 Cups has served me a huge purpose in my life, and I hope it can bring something to you too. I hope for growth in you as a reader, for personal strength, and for you to create yourself to be who you want to be. Life is short, life is hard, life is beautiful, and I love it.

So thank you for reading. Thank you for being here for me. Thank you to everyone who has supported me, loved me, and allowed me to be me. I love you all, and cheers to another 21 cups of learning and living.

To see more of my story through photos,
and for more recent updates on my recovery,
check out my website at www.21-cups.com.

I would love to hear from you!

www.ingramcontent.com/pod-product-compliance
Lightning Source LLC
Chambersburg PA
CBHW072151270326
41931CB00031B/3029
* 9 7 8 1 9 9 0 3 3 0 3 4 6 *